TALKING WITH YOUR CHILD ABOUT SEX

TALKING WITH YOUR CHILD ABOUT SEX

Questions and Answers for Children from Birth to Puberty

Dr. Mary S. Calderone
Dr. James W. Ramey

Random House · New York

Library of Congress Cataloging in Publication Data
Calderone, Mary Steichen.
Talking with your child about sex.
Bibliography: p.
Includes index.
1. Sex instruction for children. I. Ramey, James W.
II. Title.
HQ53.C34   1982   649′.65   81–48319
ISBN 0–394–52124–2   AACR2

Manufactured in the United States of America

98765432

TO

Linda		*Russell*
Francesca	our children	*Jan*
Maria		*Andy*
		Nina
Edward		
Bruce	our grandchildren	*Miles*
Edward Stuart		
Kenneth	our great-grandchildren	
Linda Joan		

and

to other children everywhere
we dedicate this book

MARY   JIM

There is something I don't know
     that I am supposed to know.
I don't know *what* it is I don't know,
     and yet am supposed to know,
and I feel I look stupid
     if I seem both not to know it
          and not know *what* it is I don't know.
Therefore I pretend I know it.
     This is nerve-racking
     since I don't know what I must pretend to know.
Therefore I pretend to know everything.

I feel you know what I am supposed to know
but you can't tell me what it is
because you don't know that I don't know what it is.

You may know what I don't know, but not
          that I don't know it,
and I can't tell you. So you will have to tell me everything.

—FROM R. D. LAING, *Knots*

PREFACE

This book has been written to help parents talk about sex with their children at each phase of their early growth and development, from infancy right up to the threshold of puberty. Sexual functioning is something all human beings share. Our kind of sexuality is unique to being human, because for us, unlike for other mammals, it involves far more than the sex act and reproduction. It involves who and what we are as male and female, how we get that way, how we feel about it and how we deal with each other about it. It also involves dreams, fantasies and ideals, and gives us pleasure, even laughter. And it involves learning, thinking, planning, postponing, developing moral values and decision-making.

A mastery of the facts of sexuality, together with a comfortable and principled set of attitudes to guide our behavior, is what we need to enjoy ourselves as sexual beings, and to respect the sexuality of others. Failing this, we can hurt ourselves and others. If we are to decrease the sexual tragedies we all know about, not only among our teenagers but also in our lives as adults, we need to learn to talk about the subject very early—easily, warmly, rationally, appropriately and, especially, lovingly—with our children.

Talking about sex is difficult for most of today's parents, whether with their children or with each other. Perhaps, as you turn the pages of this book, you'll find some surprises—maybe even some shocks. We hope that you will also find a sense of relief beginning to sweep over you—that at last the things you may have wondered or been bothered about since your own early days can be looked at with composure. As parents dig into some of these questions in an effort to help their children, maybe some of the doubts and fears and misinformation that they brought with them from their own childhoods will begin to dissipate or be seen in their true proportions. This could make it possible for the whole family to communicate more comfortably about a lot of issues that are bound to arise during the growing years, not only about sex. It is certain that when children find communication with their parents open and easy about this most difficult subject, they are enabled to move more surely and competently toward adolescence.

We think you won't want to jump in with both feet right away, but to start using this book quite slowly, testing the water here and there. If you are a parent with a first baby, it's quite simple. Start at the beginning and move ahead at your own—and the baby's—pace. But if your child is older, try to work out something that fits your special situation—perhaps dip into the chapter that matches your child's chronological age, then backtrack to find out what went just before, and then before that, and so on, back to the beginning. Then go forward again, past where your child is now, to see what happens next. How aware are you of his or her sexual interests and curiosity? Do they emerge from time to time as questions you can answer, or as questions you don't know how to answer, or feel uncomfortable about answering; or do you feel your child should not even be asking such things? All of these reactions make you a perfectly normal parent, just as your child's questions make him or her a perfectly normal child.

You don't have to push yourself in all this. As parents get more comfortable with the subject matter, the language, the facts, the knowledge that children are sexual and think sexual thoughts and do sexual things, everything about it begins to seem more natural and everyday. That's when parents begin to lose their own tensions and to make casual remarks at the right moments that tell their children that sex is an open, not closed, topic in the family. Then *everyone* begins to feel more comfortable.

Take the time to consider your child's level of sexual development. What have you noticed about how sexual words are used? What seems difficult to deal with or understand? Does your child's attitude about his or her sexuality seem positive? If you find areas that need attention, don't rush in and immediately try to catch up on everything you might have missed. It isn't necessary: Once the child knows for sure that he or she can ask you about sex just as about other things, the questions will flow naturally and can be dealt with. And remember, the same issues will come up again later, and yet again. It isn't only that children differ in the rate and evenness of their development; it's also that with the big topics like reproduction, each retelling is a chance to add a new nugget of knowledge. After all, even though you've had a child, you yourself are probably still learning new things about the process.

Try to be alert to how your child approaches and reacts to sexual topics. Is there anything in the child's behavior or attitude that seems to require your attention? You may sense a need for help that the child can't seem to put into words. Or a situation may have arisen with a playmate that tells you your child needs support and comfort. Parents who are aware can often meet and resolve an issue before it becomes a problem.

Although talking with children about sex is traditionally "mother's responsibility," in families with fathers present this can (and should, we think) be a shared responsibility for both parents. Letting mothers do it all serves only to cheat both children and fathers of the great adventure and joy of involvement of the *whole* family in this important enterprise.

Both parents, in their quiet moments together, will find it rewarding to share and compare their own earliest sexual memories. Remembering how it was growing up can bring clarifying insights. How old were you? What happened? Was someone else involved? What did you do? What did they do? Who said what? How did it all turn out? How do you feel about it now? Working through these situations can be very useful. It can also be healing if what happened, remembered as hurtful, can now be looked at in a more rational light. If, as a child, you were taken advantage of by someone more powerful than yourself, a clarification and validation of your anger can be part of the healing.

Talking with your partner about your own childhood sexual experiences should make it easier to find an opportunity to initiate a similar discussion with your child. You might even find that telling your child about your own sexual experience when you were his or her age will free your child to talk about sex with you. If there is no response, it might be because the child doesn't quite believe you *are* open to questions, or isn't interested because he or she is not ready for the topic, or is bored because the topic already seems like an old story. Try again another day just to prove that you are askable.

There are lots of different ways you might arrange to have a talk with your child. Sometimes topics about the physical body and sexuality—and our attitudes about these things—come up most easily when you are in skin-to-skin contact: lap sitting, back rubbing or just snuggled together on a sofa. Sometimes you will want to sit down together for a heart-to-heart talk, making eye contact to keep a closeness with each other. And sometimes it may be easiest to talk casually while you work side by side, folding laundry or finishing the dinner cleanup, partly diverted by the handwork you are doing so that the child can control the approach to subjects that seem very sensitive to him or her.

Here are some general comments about the process of such discussions, with suggestions that we find helpful:

(1) Don't try to initiate a discussion when your mind is on preparing dinner or meeting a deadline. You wouldn't start a serious conversation with an adult under such circumstances, and your child deserves as much attention as anyone else. Be careful not to lecture. Remember, you're trying to start a conversation, during which it is probably even more important that you listen than that you talk. Pick a time when the two of you (or three of you if both parents are present) are alone, and not likely to be interrupted. Some deep feelings come out slowly and thoughts have to be given plenty of chance to develop.

(2) Make sure you give recognition to a good line of thought that shows your child is really dealing with the issues. Respond positively even if you are criticized; try to emphasize the good growing-up kinds of things, and take the negative ones in stride by suggesting or emphasizing how they might be better.

(3) Set clear rules that fit family patterns. Discuss how to change the rules, when that seems to be needed.

(4) Be encouraging about behavior that is appropriate or shows maturation. "Goodness" and "badness" are not very helpful in dealing with sexual functions; "appropriate" is a more sensitive word to use, as it leaves room for change and growth.

(5) When you've handled something well, let yourself feel good about it.

Once you've broken the ice, each subsequent discussion will be easier. Gradually a pattern will develop that works comfortably and suits *your* family's needs.

This book is equally applicable to the traditional two-parent family, to the single-parent home, to the home where a child is being raised by grandparents, to a household with several adults or to unmarried parents or caretakers. Though we often speak here about both parents, we know that growing up in a single-parent home need not have adverse effects on the sexual growth and development of children. Sometimes single mothers are hesitant about this, but there's no reason to worry about it. All children need their mother's hugs and strokes. There is much more risk in depriving children of physical affection.

When children of divorced parents get into trouble, the difficulty usually lies not in the singleness of the parent but in the fact that most divorced mothers have a lowered standard of living, may have to live in a poor and rough neighborhood or are subject to other similarly undesirable living circumstances.

A child is born sexual, a trait just as characteristic of being human as the inborn capacities to walk upright and to speak. We delightedly welcome and help the children to develop their ability to walk and talk, but the same is not true of this other aspect of the child's humanness, his or her inborn capacity for simple sexual pleasure. Yet this too requires adult guidance and support for its healthy evolution.

This need for guidance and support may be *the* crucial barrier for you as a parent to overcome. Once you can understand and accept your child's sexuality as right and normal and beautiful in its potentialities—the same as all your child's other endowments— then you will be free to move toward helping the child in his/her sexual socialization.

Consider how we socialize other natural functions—eating, for instance: We are happy if our child has a good appetite; we are proud when the child picks up the spoon for the first time instead of plunging a fist into the cereal bowl. Later it will be the niceties of fork, knife and napkin, of sitting at the family table and joining in the family conversation that we will applaud. Still later will come learning how to behave in a restaurant. What you are teaching here regarding food is not "good" or "bad" ways to eat, but appropriateness of eating behavior.

We have just described the socialization of eating as a primary life function. So also there is socialization of sexual pleasure as a primary life function. Remember that reproduction will not be possible until around twelve years of age. In those first twelve years you will want to teach your child the meanings of sexual pleasure in his or her life—gradually, in small amounts, related to appropriateness and responsibility—in readiness for puberty.

As a result of our work in this field and after long and careful examination of the research of others and of the conclusions reached by eminent child specialists, it has become clear to us that society must cease trying to interfere with the child's natural discovery and enjoyment of self-pleasuring. There is no need for verbal or even nonverbal disapproval of pleasure. Instead we should give clear signals of "okays" that will lead to the acceptance and enjoyment of sexual behavior that is appropriate to the child's stage of development. By doing so we will promote a healthy, positive sexuality and help spare our children the many sexual problems that today's adults experience.

There is no need to be discouraged if these thoughts are new to you. It may even be that your child is older and you fear you may already have "damaged" him or her. Don't be fearful of this, for human beings have the most remarkable capacities for getting well. Take your time about it. Talk with your partner, with trusted friends or a counselor. As you gain knowledge, your attitudes about your own sexuality will probably become more open and accepting, and you will find you are able to feel and act spontaneously toward your children in such ways that healing and normal sexual development can take place.

You will also find it much easier to teach your child the basic religious or moral values to which your family subscribes by accepting and honoring your child's erotic potential, instead of denying him or her the right to sexual pleasure. When you do this, you are building respect for yourselves, for each other, and for the life energies of each member of your family.

In return your children will feel secure in what you have made possible for them, especially of your trust in the worth of their sexuality and in their growing ability to manage it appropriately and responsibly. Adolescence will not come upon them like a storm to knock them off their foundations. Instead they will be prepared for it by the sense of family unity, security and love that we all seek and cherish.

ACKNOWLEDGMENTS

We wish to thank Lorna Brown for seeing the merit in this project, finding it a home and providing continuous support.

We also wish to acknowledge the thoughtful, encouraging help of Mary Howell, who took time out from her busy schedule to provide a reassuring outsider's perspective on the material.

We are especially grateful to Charlotte Mayerson, our editor. Her skills, cooperation, patience and friendship saw us through the task of completing this book.

Finally, we greatly value the support of Betty Ramey, who believed in the project from the beginning.

CONTENTS

TALKING
WITH YOUR
CHILD ABOUT
SEX

1

The Newborn and
the First Eighteen Months

It surprises us to be reminded that in ancient as well as medieval times, European children were allowed to be openly sexual, and that in many non-Western cultures this is still the case. In the sixteenth century, however, Europeans began to redefine the child as "innocent," meaning that before it reached puberty, the child was not considered a sexual being. We have retained this belief into modern times.

A principal source of the idea that small children are not sexual comes from the view of sex as "dirty" or "wicked." In addition, though most of us are aware that sexuality is a source of pleasure, we also recognize that sex is *used* in our society for profit and oppression—as in advertising, entertainment, prostitution, pornography, sexual slavery of women and children, and the like. We rightfully and understandably do not want to think that our young children could have any connection with a world that so viciously exploits women and youth in the pandering of sexual services.

In our wish to protect our children from that unsavory aspect of adult life, we "forget to remember" the intimate, private and personal pleasures of sexuality as part of the goodness of life. To know oneself as a sexual being is, first and foremost, to respect, honor and appreciate one's own body. Children—and babies— spontaneously begin this process of self-knowing, which must be developed if sexuality is to be a vital ingredient in a mature relationship between adults.

This view of infant sexuality has been slow to take hold. We have only gradually been willing, in the last half-century, to acknowledge that normal children truly are sexual. Professionals who study children have recently affirmed the strong sexuality of the newborn.

To begin to understand these findings, let's look at some of the ways that we use the words "sexual" and "sexuality." First of all, these terms are used to talk about the awareness that one *is* male or female. Does the infant know that? Of course not. Yet every normal baby will know it by the time he or she is two and certainly not later than three, when *he* will associate himself with men and boys, and *she* with girls and women. How does that happen? From the beginning, quite unconsciously, parents and everyone else treat a baby quite differently depending upon whether it is a girl or a boy. In addition, males are attracted to males and females to females—like to like—by a process of elemental psychological identification that includes such chemical factors as smell. This active identification by the child with others of its own gender, along with the direct and indirect teaching of others, provides the cues by which the child learns its *gender identity*.

Another aspect of this male/female training is that every society has its own standards as to the *kinds* of men and women it wants its children to grow into. Mothers and fathers the world over start very early in the child's development to impress on it just how it should behave if it is a girl or a boy. This is the way that children learn their *gender roles*; that is, they learn not only whether they are male or female (*gender identity*), they also learn what is expected of members of their sex.

The standards of gender role training are quite arbitrary in each social group, and are subject to arbitrary change, for there is nothing biologically inevitable about how a man or a woman *should* act. In our society, gender role expectations have changed a great deal in the past few decades. We have also become a more pluralistic society, so that there are many varied patterns for being an acceptable male or female, depending partly on what countries our parents or grandparents came from, partly on which sections of the United States we live in, partly on our social and economic class, level of education and life philosophy.

The third factor of sexuality is sexual feelings, and the actions taken in response to those feelings. Though parents often cannot imagine how their young baby could even have sexual feelings, the fact is that they do. For example, in most male infants, erections are seen at or soon after birth. The analogue in a baby girl, an erect clitoris, is not so easy to observe, but the vaginal lubrication that accompanies clitoral erection can be seen just after birth, lasting each time from several seconds to a few minutes. Periodic penile and clitoral erection and periodic vaginal lubrication continue throughout life, and both occur in sexual arousal. Furthermore, very young babies have been noted by competent observers to experience what could only be interpreted as orgasm, and they learn after a few months how deliberately to produce this kind of pleasure for themselves.

How can an intelligent society continue to deny what is—and always has been—so plainly there? Worse, how can we permit ourselves to go on not only denying it but punishing it, trying to stop it, calling it "bad" or "sinful"? How can a baby be bad or sinful for doing what he or she was created to do—learn how to walk, to talk, to think and how to explore and civilize his or her inborn sexuality?

Throughout childhood boys and girls learn to know and experience their own bodies, each with its own unique sexual repertoire. This is the only way they can grow to understand, in later years, that sex can be a component in a mutually respectful, loving relationship. The ability to share sexual intimacy with another person and to make intelligent use of our own reproductive potential requires that you behave responsibly toward your partner as well as yourself. Full and open opportunity throughout childhood is essential for such awareness and such a capacity to be developed.

Because this chapter is especially for new parents and parents-to-be, we have presented some questions and answers to help them (or other adults who are in charge of growing infants) to expand their knowledge about infant sexuality so that they will be able to recognize, follow, help and feel comfortable about the sexual development of the infants under their care.

The remainder of this book is based on the assumption that you intend to accept your child's sexuality as the fact it is, that you want to build on it rather than destroy or cripple it and that you are willing to put time and energy into learning how to do so.

What are some of the things to watch for to help me keep track of my baby's normal sexual development?

The early development of sexuality is founded in two kinds of experiences. The first is being held, fondled, caressed—learning about the *sensuality* of the body's covering. Skin-to-skin contact is an important part of this learning—when the baby is at the breast, or naked after a bath or at clothes-changing time, or when you simply want to share that experience with him or her. Babies should have plenty of opportunities to cuddle with others in addition to their mothers: fathers, grandparents, older siblings, anyone who has the time and energy to be a loving caretaker.

Whether the baby is nursing or bottle-fed, feeding time is cuddle time. If your baby is a boy you may notice his automatic and normal response of erection. There is no need to stimulate or encourage this—it happens. The important thing is not to *dis*courage or interfere with it.

A baby girl's response is clitoral erection, which you are less likely to notice. It is usually accompanied by vaginal lubrication; this can be quite copious, so it's nice if you know enough not to worry about it.

There may be times when the baby becomes intensely self-absorbed. The infant's body will stiffen, then relax, then stiffen again. The face and body may flush and the child will react quite negatively if interrupted. Occasionally there might be grunting, which you may think means a bowel movement, yet none comes. This may well be orgasm, which has been observed even in the early weeks of life. That's normal, too, for many boy and girl babies. Self-exploration of their body parts and responses will come later as the second kind of experience that is basic to healthy early sexual development.

It is much easier for a baby girl to bring herself to orgasm by squeezing her thighs together because of the way her vulva and clitoris are positioned. Boys will catch up after a few months, when they have developed sufficient coordination to find their penises with their hands.

Many children masturbate before age one, without their parents recognizing what is happening. We assume that nearly all babies, both girls and boys, learn this way of pleasuring themselves in the first year of life.

I'm expecting my first child soon. How can I get the baby off to the best start?

You and the baby will do it together—along with the baby's father and/or others (such as housemates, grandparents, lovers and friends) who want to be close to the infant.

As soon after delivery as possible the naked child can be placed right in your arms—usually this may be done before the umbilical cord is cut. You can hold the baby against your breast where he or she can feel the warmth of your skin and hear your heartbeat, which has been a steady companion for the past nine months. Soon she or he can nurse for the first time and get to know the lovely, distinctive smell of your milk and your skin. You and the baby can have your first long looks at each other.

Newborns can, and need to, fix their eyes on the faces of their mothers and other significant persons. They will look intently for long periods of time. You should talk to the baby, so that voices become familiar as well as faces.

All this can take place while the afterbirth is coming, even if you have some local anesthesia. This first close intimate contact, in the early minutes and hours of the baby's life, with the mother and other significant persons, is called "bonding." The baby bonds to the others, and they bond to the infant, creating a primitive, mystical and wonderful attachment that will be important as a cornerstone of later relationships. This bonding experience will be repeated many times over the first few months of the baby's life—although probably never with such meaningful intensity as during the first minutes and hours after the baby's birth. It is important for you in accepting the baby into your life, and for the baby in creating a trustworthy world of caretakers.

Babies who are born by Caesarean section can be given to their mothers immediately, as with babies born by vaginal delivery. If the baby is born prematurely or for some other reason has to be watched closely in a special nursery, arrangements can—and should—be made for the mother or parents to be with the baby frequently, for the skin and eye and voice contact that are the ingredients of bonding.

What has all this to do with sexuality? Everything. It is through bonding that a sense of trust begins to be established as the basis for the good feelings that will continue to develop between the new baby and those who take care of her or him. The capacity for intimacy and trust established in infancy will be echoed years later in the capacity for intimacy and trust in a love relationship.

Is there any difference in subsequent sexual development between breast- and bottle-fed babies?

There often is but there needn't be. Breast-feeding ensures close physical contact and supports the baby's trust, emotional security and natural eroticism as part of the feeding process. If the infant is to be bottle-fed, it is important for its emotional development that the mother hold the baby close against her breast, talking to it and maintaining eye and voice contact during the feeding. When the bottle is always given to it in this way, the emotional results for the baby should be the same as with breast-feeding.

My little boy is just a few weeks old, but ever since his birth I've had dreams that seem pretty strange to me. I dream about him as a male, not as just my baby, and I seem turned on in these dreams. Is there something wrong with me?

This kind of erotic reaction to a baby is not unusual, especially with first boys. After all, here you are, at a moment when your glandular system is going through a period of intense readjustment after nine months of profound changes due to pregnancy. The pregnancy itself brought with it powerful emotions, as did the experience of birth. Your sexual relationship with your husband may have been changed by the pregnancy—–you may find yourself *less* interested or *more* interested in sex than usual.

Then too, you are being confronted several times a day by this tiny stranger with whose genital organs you must deal in a most intimate manner. And you are also witnessing entirely normal erections.

All in all, your reactions are not surprising and should not disturb you. Just as your physiological system will readjust itself so will your psychological self. Eventually you will come to see your baby for what he is—your son—and you will have adjusted to the whole business. Your erotic fantasies should then stop bothering you. Remember, though, that fantasies are just that—fantasies. They are harmless as long as they remain so, and you do not act on them.

And speaking realistically, we can offer you a prophetic word of wisdom: Perhaps fifteen years from now you may find yourself having similar feelings about a suddenly tall, handsome young male—your son! Remember then that none of us need hold ourselves responsible for our feelings, but only for what we do about them: If not responded to inappropriately, they are entirely harmless.

I always feel sexually stimulated when the baby nurses. Could that overstimulate the baby?

No, it wouldn't affect the baby as long as you were quiet and peaceful while it was nursing. Many mothers experience this feeling —it's quite a usual thing.

Why are girl and boy babies so different, right from the start?

There are, of course, some inborn differences between the sexes— although, in general, there is more variability among all boys and among all girls than *between* all boys and all girls. But most adults start right at birth to treat male and female infants differently. Mothers who use both pink and blue baby clothes have noticed how differently people react to the infant if it is dressed in the "wrong" color. This difference in the way we respond tends to reinforce whatever inborn differences there are, and thus begins the process of socializing the child into what is considered proper behavior for males and females.

Why do babies get erections while nursing?

The mouth is an important part of a marvelous complex of nerve connections that make up the human sexual response system. Other parts of that system include the skin, the eyes, the sense of taste and smell, and the genital organs. All are linked with the sexual center in the brain where pleasure is felt—whether the baby is male or female.

The baby learns almost immediately after birth to recognize its mother by the taste and smell of her nipple and breast as well as by the sight of her face and the sound of her voice. These then become linked to the satisfaction of nursing, being fed and held close and feeling the mother's warm skin. These sensations are transmitted upward to the conscious part of the brain and, via other connections, to the sexual center which perceives them as pleasurable. All of this happens in an instant, and erection is automatic because of the very direct nerve linkage between the pleasure center and the penis or clitoris. The erect penis is easy to notice in an unclothed baby. It is less easy to see the erect clitoris, but we can notice the wetness of vaginal lubrication. These are all indications of normal infant sexual response.

We were told baby should have skin-to-skin contact with the father, too, and our baby loves lying on her father's chest. But I've noticed that my husband often seems to want to make love with me after that happens. Isn't that rather strange?

Many things can lead to sexual desire—things seen, heard, smelled, tasted, touched or fantasized. Being with a new baby is an exciting new experience for both you and your husband. Sexual arousal is a quite normal reaction to such intimate skin-to-skin contact between the baby and your husband—as is his desire to make love with *you*.

When I smooth mineral oil on the baby's body after his bath, or when changing him, he often gets an erection. Will it do any harm if I smooth his erection with the oil too?

Because of the pleasure network of nerve connections, it's natural for an erection to accompany skin massage. Obviously too, when bathing, smoothing on oil, changing diapers or cleansing the baby's bottom, your fingers quite naturally will touch his penis and an erection may result. This does no harm at all and it is not necessary to avoid it. Girl babies are similarly stimulated to have clitoral erections. It's possible that more than casual touching might introduce an artificial element of stimulation, and since we know little or nothing about the effects of such touching, we feel that the healthiest way is simply to let the natural thing happen, without either encouraging or discouraging it. By six or seven months, in any case, the little boy will himself be in charge and able to begin his own sexual life by masturbating when he feels like it, just as girl babies do often at an earlier age.

Isn't it really the mother's job to hold and feed and comfort the baby? My wife does it so well, and after all, men don't really know about those things. I'm very nervous about holding him.

The doubts you express are familiar to many first-time fathers, maybe because they often don't have a long enough opportunity right after the baby's birth to bond with the baby. You may not yet see him/her as a *person* who counts in *your* life as importantly as in your wife's life. Try taking over a little more care of the baby every day. When he wakes up for a feeding, you do the picking up and the changing, smiling and talking to him in a low voice all the time to hold his attention. You might even hold off the feeding until he starts fussing for it. Keep your eyes and attention fixed on him, hold him against your bare chest and stroke the skin of his bare body. If he's on the bottle, try to give him at least one bottle every day. You will become more and more close and important to each other.

Soon he will begin to look for you. You might even be lucky enough to catch his very first smile of recognition. None of you three should ever feel you have to compete for love and attention. There is plenty of each for all of you, and sharing one another's love is how you become a family.

We live in a one-bedroom apartment. How long can we continue to have sex while the baby is in the room?

If you and your young baby share a room, you shouldn't worry about having sex unless it disturbs the baby's sleep. That is, you shouldn't worry more about the effects on the baby of being in the same room when you have sex than about the effects of your talking or laughing or singing in the same room with the sleeping baby. If the baby wakes and has to be quieted, that would interrupt your lovemaking as well as the baby's sleep. But if the young baby did wake and lie quietly, perhaps watching, while the parents made love, there would be no adverse effects; perhaps there would even be good effects for the baby—to experience the energy of love and caring.

There is a lot of difference of opinion about children seeing their parents in sexual intercourse. Many families throughout the world still share sleeping quarters, as was done in our own recent past. However, until we know more about possible consequences, most parents may want to play safe about this and to set about two years of age as the time when lovemaking will be done in private. Each family will need to consider its own circumstances and feelings in this matter. Just remember, babies and young children have a marvelous capacity for adapting to circumstances. Even in a small apartment, of course, it is always possible to roll the baby's crib to a hallway or another room, even behind a screen at the other side of the room, to create something like separate sleeping places for baby and parents. Usually, everybody sleeps more restfully this way.

I've noticed our three-week-old daughter sometimes has quite a discharge on her vulva. It even dries to a crust once in a while. Is there something wrong?

Baby girls begin their sexual lives with lubrication of the vagina immediately after birth. It is exactly the same reaction as in sexual response, and accompanies clitoral erection. Erections and lubrication of the vagina will continue throughout life. Vaginal mucus also occurs periodically as part of a monthly pattern and, in mature women, change in amount and type of discharge can be used to monitor fertility.

While a vaginal discharge is normally to be expected, the amount can vary from almost invisible to one that covers the vaginal opening. When the discharge dries, it can make a thin crusting, but this should not alarm you unless there are signs of irritation, such as redness or a rash. You can soften the crusted discharge with warm water and it will come right off, and you can talk about it with your pediatrician on the next visit.

It's hard to get used to having our baby boy spray my face or clothing with urine while I'm changing or cleansing him. What can I do?

Lots of parents feel like this, so keep several things in mind. First, be sure not to startle the baby by jumping or shouting if this happens. Instead, *smile*! Second, remember that urine has no bacteria or other "bad things." It is approximately $99\frac{99}{100}$ percent plain water with some salts added. Third, remember that the erect penis cannot urinate—and vice versa. Because the baby's penis gets naturally erect from light touching, changing and cleansing acts as a kind of insurance against water damage. Remember as you clean the rest of his body to lay a fresh diaper or washcloth lightly over the penis, like an umbrella, to catch the spray.

Won't leaving the baby naked promote masturbation?

It won't "promote" it, it will simply permit it to happen—as it will with every baby who has the opportunity to develop naturally. Allowing the baby to discover and practice masturbation is healthy. Interference or attempts to interfere with masturbation can cause strong feelings of resistance, anger or frustration. These feelings may carry over into and disturb adult sexual life years later. Most experts in the psychology of development (and most therapists) look upon sexual self-pleasuring as a natural and inevitable part of human development that should not be interfered with. As the child grows older, he or she can be made aware of the importance of masturbating only in appropriate circumstances. (See Chapters 2 and 3.)

If the baby touches his or her genitals and then sticks those fingers in his or her mouth, what about germs?

You don't have to be afraid of the baby's own germs, for he or she is immune to these. Anyway, if the baby's bottom has been cleansed after its bowel movement, then its genitals are probably as clean as its mouth!

My friend says if you cater to a baby by holding it too much, it will get spoiled. Is that true?

Just the opposite. Remember, a baby is totally helpless. If it is allowed to "cry it out," it learns that it *cannot* depend on someone to respond to its felt needs: for changing a wet diaper, or for hunger, or burping, or simply for company and play and warmth and security. If these needs are not met, then what may be interfered with is growing up into a trusting, dependable person able to enter into and sustain loving relationships.

My aunt says I should begin toilet training right away and get it over with, but my baby is only four months old. Isn't that sort of early?

Yes, much too early, because toilet training isn't something you do *to* your baby but *with* your baby when she or he is ready. The more relaxed you can be about toilet training, the easier it will be for you. Then you will be alert to catch the signals your baby will surely give you when, in due time, he or she is ready to take charge of this particular function.

If I try to smile pleasantly while changing my little girl's dirty diapers, won't it be more difficult to toilet-train her later?

Just the opposite, really, provided you can learn to see the urine and feces of your baby for what they are—body products that prove that someone important to you is healthy. Later on, usually around two, the baby will show in different ways when she is ready to take charge of her own body elimination. The toilet training will be easier and faster if you haven't mixed in your own feelings of distaste with what should be the baby's growing sense of pleasure and self-command. As she learns how to dispose of her body products in appropriate ways that earn your approval, you two can share your good feelings.

How soon should I go about naming the body parts to the baby?

Most parents start naming the parts of the body before the baby actually understands what is going on, because both grownups and babies love the game. The important thing is to include the genitals, giving them no more or less emphasis than any other part, and using their correct names. Most mothers and fathers enjoy turning the naming into a game, touching each part and saying, "What's that?" and then giving the answer: "That's your hair, or nose or eyes, or bellybutton, or vulva, or anus or penis." Try going down (or up) the body in sequence. As the baby develops, you can ask, "Where's your nose?" or "your toes?" or "your vulva?" and the child will clutch the part with pleasure at knowing the answer. When talking begins, you can go back to pointing and asking, "What's that?" and wait for the answer. This is always a happy, laughing, learning game if all names of all body parts are learned with equal facility and composure.

My husband found our three-year-old, Tommy, exploring the baby's vulva. He took Tommy's hand away but then pointed out and named the baby's sexual parts. Shouldn't he have punished Tommy instead?

Your son's curiosity as to how the baby's genitals are different from his own is normal, and your husband reacted positively. Even though Tommy is still too young to understand completely, his father satisfied his curiosity while, at the same time, indicating that direct touching was inappropriate. And he did not make the boy feel guilty or ashamed for having done something that he could not possibly have thought was bad.

No doubt your son will have to repeat this inspection of his little sister a number of times before he satisfies his curiosity, just as she will later want to inspect him. Then they will surely both want to talk about their different body parts. All this is common with all children. (See Chapters 2 and 3.)

Shouldn't you avoid overstimulating an infant? I think my friend must have done that with her son because, by ten months, he would hold on to her and thrust against her with his pelvis.

Most boy and girl babies, when they learn to stand up, enjoy hugging and closeness with parents. Pelvic movements and rubbing the body against another person are natural and should not be looked upon as any more disturbing than nuzzling or stroking or licking with the tongue—something many babies enjoy at a certain stage. We adults tend to read our own feelings into what is happening, and from our adult perspective we may relate such pelvic thrusting to intercourse. The baby doesn't make that connection at all, but simply has good feelings from the closeness with his mother. Soon, the baby will be old enough to understand from the parents what ways of showing affection are appropriate, and with whom.

Is there any way I can tell if my baby is getting enough affection?

It's easier to tell when there is *not* enough affection. When parent-infant relationships are not warm enough, infants tend to withdraw into their own world. They tend not to react to other people in the smiling, responsive way that is typical of an infant with affectionate and demonstrative parents. It is significant that an infant who doesn't get enough affection seldom engages in genital play. Children who receive enough affection develop normally, and *genital play is always present*. It's as if the capacity for sexual pleasure and the interest and skill of the infant in producing it are indicators of the general well-being of the baby. There is a close parallel with food: We all understand that the vigor and appetite with which a baby eats is a measure of health. It is the same with sex.

2

Eighteen
Months to Three Years

In only eighteen months the child has changed from a helpless infant into an active toddler. He or she has already learned many things: Instead of crying, for example, speech is now used to get wants filled, and the beginnings of a vocabulary are already in place. He or she can walk, run and climb, and, as to eating, has moved to baby foods and then to the family table. More time is now spent awake than asleep, and the child's world has expanded from bassinet to crib to playpen—and from being carried—to the present free run of the family living space.

Social horizons have expanded too. The child is now aware of people other than parents—an older brother or sister perhaps, grandparents or friends who are frequent visitors, a babysitter. He or she also has other more casual acquaintances—the postal carrier, grocery clerk, butcher, police officer. Experience and information are flooding in, and they require a process of continuous sorting out for the toddler's most immediate task: *me*. The child is constantly on the move—learning, doing and investigating—in the natural drive to become independent and autonomous. The theme is me, myself, I can do it.

From a year and a half to three, several areas of experience will affect the development of the child's sexuality. By age two, the child has become more or less aware that various things are being expected of him or her. One of these is that the body products to which the child has strong feelings of attachment are now supposed to be put into a certain place at a certain time. Urinating and having bowel movements can no longer just happen. In short, toilet training has begun.

In our society, toilet training commonly results in some conflict between parent and child. To avoid this, it is important that it not be something that you do *to* the baby against the baby's will. Instead it should be a learning experience *for* him or her, when it appears that the child is ready for it. This is somewhere around two years, but the child will let you know that she or he is ready by grunting, by gesturing, by running toward the potty chair, by holding on to his or her genitals or in any other of a number of ways you can learn to recognize. Usually you and the child will come to use a particular word or syllable that means "I have to use the toilet now."

Young children experience pleasure when urinating or having a bowel movement, and may want to play with their urine or feces. They also enjoy examining their own or each other's genitals. Don't be surprised or upset to find the child doing either or both on the potty chair. The experimenting is normal, and as to the cleanliness issues, remember that the child is immune to his or her own germs. Anyway, you will be teaching about hand-washing after using the potty.

The language and words used about sex and body functions vary greatly from home to home. All children have a nose, ears, arms, feet, fingers and toes, but often boys have a wee-wee, a peter, a thing, instead of a penis. And what most girls have, if anything, is described as "down there" or "down below," instead of being called what it is—a vulva. And the important things contained *within* the vulva (clitoris, urethra or peehole, and vagina) seem to have to exist without any kind of name. Recent efforts toward enlightenment in this matter have focused on naming the vagina, which is not, in fact, the most sensitive and active part of the female genitals. That part—the part that the child is *most* likely to experience and want to know about—is the clitoris. It is as if we have wanted to oversimplify the female genitalia, labeling them all as "vagina."

Deliberate adult avoidance of the area between waist and knees can hardly be expected to go unnoticed by the child, especially when other body parts are freely mentioned. Since the child already knows that this is an important pleasure center of the body, such avoidance can cause confusion and lay the groundwork for later problems.

Body contact with parents has been a meaningful and important part of the child's life up to now, but during this period he or she may experience a quite sudden lessening of this contact. This is especially true with boys. Notice how in playgrounds, mothers tend to push their toddler boys away from them at younger ages than they do their toddler girls. The body contact of fathers with their boys of two to four tends to become roughhouse style—feinting, tickling, punching—whereas with daughters of the same age both fathers and mothers tend to continue tender cuddling and hugging. Yet small boys and small girls are quite alike in their needs: Both like to show their strong affection for parents, other children, family pets and cuddly toys by much hugging and kissing. They want to be stroked and hugged and kissed in return by the people in their lives. Rocking and singing to a young child means body closeness and security. Changing the pattern too suddenly "now that you're a big boy (or girl) of three" can bewilder a child and interrupt the smooth growth of self-acceptance and feelings of worth.

At the same time, the child is struggling with social questions that have a bearing on his or her sexual training. In many families wearing clothes becomes an issue, along with learning family rules about closed bathroom or bedroom doors, and about touching others, especially adults. Even a strange visitor may pinch or pat the toddler, but reciprocation is usually not allowed, and touching his or her own body is now subject to changes in rules: What may be done in the bathtub may not be allowed in the living room. What is allowed in the living room may not be allowed away from home. How a family formulates these social rules for the child often depends on what the parents themselves were taught in early childhood, even though that training may not fit the kind of sexual world in which the children are growing up.

Finally there is the question of sex pleasure. Facing up to its existence still causes great unease to many parents. To see a toddler fondling his penis is hard for some parents to accept with equanimity. And to watch and accept a tiny girl's self-pleasuring is almost impossible for many parents to accept. Many people feel that little girls, even more than little boys, should be "pure," which is to say they should not be interested in sex at all. This is only one of many instances of the double standard we have for our children.

The pleasure children get from masturbation should not just be ignored. It should be clearly and positively acknowledged by their parents. Otherwise the children's self-respect, as well as their immense capacity for logical thinking and action, is hampered. "I'm glad it feels good to touch your clitoris (or penis). That's the way it is meant to feel." Just as your first step as a parent or caretaker was to accept that children *are* sexual (Chapter 1), now your big step is accepting *how* children are sexual. This then brings you into direct confrontation with the issue of self-pleasuring, or masturbation, and that may be very uncomfortable for you, depending on how you were treated in this regard by *your* parents and peers. You may not even remember actual occurrences, but they may have gone something like this: "That's '*bad*' " (or "*dirty*" or "*sinful*"). "Don't let me catch you doing it again!" Out of fear you obeyed: You never again let an adult "catch" you. But did it stop you? If it didn't, how did you feel about the repetition that you yourself knew was inevitable? And the sense of guilt? If it did stop you, what has been the effect on your own adult sexual life?

Focusing too harshly on toilet training or not allowing the child to freely touch his or her own body sets up confusion about who actually owns the body. It also sends the message that some parts of the child's body are bad. Instead, we should convey, "Your body is lovely and good—and it's *yours*." "You can learn how to manage it and we are happy to help you" is the message to be conveyed by the parents' attitudes.

The mother who carefully interposes a washcloth between her hand and her baby's body is not giving the important message that little boys and girls may learn to clean their whole bodies, including the penis or vulva, with their own hands in a gentle, intimate and loving way.

Masturbation adds to your understanding of your body and your pleasure in the way it functions. It can also serve to comfort you, as a temporary way of dealing with frustrations and disappointments until they can be resolved in practical ways. The child knows very well that sex *feels* good. Associating badness or dirtiness with it creates inner conflict impossible for him or her to resolve.

If you succeed in completely repressing your child's masturbation, he or she may substitute bed-wetting, finger-sucking or nail-biting. More important, by stunting the child's sexual development, you may be creating problems for his or her later development into an aware, responsible person who appreciates sexual experience in a mature relationship.

Most children are not going to stop masturbating just because their parents tell them to—it gives them too much pleasure and their need is too great. What may happen, however, is that children who have been scolded or who have sensed their parents' unspoken disapproval will feel they are disobeying or acting badly when they masturbate. Their self-esteem may be damaged, and they may feel confused or guilty. Perhaps they will incorporate their parents' displeasure into the experience itself.

Since sexual capacity is present from birth, learning to use it competently and responsibly must go along with learning to use one's other endowments of body and mind. Children invariably learn sexual facts, attitudes and behavior from their parents between birth and age three, regardless of what parents think or do about it. If you are aware of this, you have a great opportunity to make sure that whatever learning takes place will be positive. You can support your child in the development of his or her sexuality with the same volition and skill you teach bowel control, language ability and muscle coordination.

What's that?

It's called a breast.

Why don't I have any?

For girls: You do, right here, but it's very small and flat. When you get much bigger, you will have breasts that stick out.

For boys: You do, right here. It's just very small and flat.

What's that?

That's my nipple. And look, you have nipples too.

They're little.

For girls: They'll be bigger when you're bigger and get breasts.

For boys: They'll be bigger when you're bigger, but only grown-up women have big breasts. Men's breasts stay small and flat.

What's that?

That's a penis.

What's it for?

That's what boys pee with.

Look, it stands up.

That's right; all penises do that sometimes.

Daddy's got a penis too?

Yes, all men and boys do.

It stands up too?

Sometimes. It feels good that way.

What's that?

It's called a vulva.

Why is it all hairy?

All grown-up women have hair there.

Why don't I?

For girls: That's because you're not grown up. When you are, you'll have hair there, just like Mommy.

For boys: You'll have hair around your penis when you grow up.

What's that little bag? It's lumpy.

That's a scrotum, and the two round lumps like little balls are called testicles.

Why doesn't our new baby have a penis like me?

For boys: Because she's a girl, and pees from a different place. Her urine comes out of her peehole, which is in her vulva. Boys like you have penises to urinate with. Girls and boys are made differently.

What's that on our new baby? I don't have one like that.

For girls: That's a penis, and that's where his urine comes out. Girls' urine comes out from a different place, right there in the vulva. You can see it when you urinate. Girls and boys are made differently.

What's down here between my legs?

For girls: That's called your vulva. There are important parts inside your vulva.

How can I see it?

Sit down and spread your legs. Now you hold this mirror, and I'll turn on the flashlight. There at the top—that's your clitoris. Next is your peehole, where your urine comes out. Next is your vagina. That's where a baby could come out someday when you are grown up, if you want to have one.

What do you call way down here?

That's your anus, where you push your bowel movement out. See how close it is to your vulva, where your vagina and peehole are? They are clean, but your bowel movement has germs in it that can cause sickness. That's why you should wipe your anus after a BM, from front to back, like this. That way BM can't get up here, where it could make your vagina or peehole sore. Then we always wash our hands after we wipe so they will be clean for certain.

What's this bump?

That's your clitoris.

What's it for?

For feeling good when you touch it, like your brother's penis. That feels good, too, when he makes it stand up.

Does mine stand up?

Yes, it does, but it's hard to see. And it *feels* good. All girls are made that way.

Mommy too?

Mommy too, and your sister.

Daddy too?

No, Daddy is made like your brother. Everybody is like girls or like boys. But remember, making yourself feel good by touching your clitoris or penis is for when you're alone, in your room, with the door closed. Everybody feels private about that, and likes it better that way. I do.

Daddy too?

Yes, Daddy too. When you see our door closed, please don't come in.

My sister too?

Yes, everybody.

And my little brother?

Well, he's littler than you, so he doesn't know about privacy yet. When he's bigger, you can teach him that when the door is closed that means that someone wants to be private.

Why can't I pee in the bath water?

Because toilets are for peeing and bathtubs are for bathing. If you want to pee in the bathtub, do it *before* we run the bath water. People like to bathe in plain water, not in pee-water.

Why can't I play with my urine?

Your urine is nice and clean when it comes out of you, but if it gets on your clothes or on the floor, after a while it leaves a smell that people don't like.

Why is a BM dirty?

It has lots of germs in it. The germs are our friends and they do good work for us when they are in our body. But our germs are not good for other people and they make our BM smell. So we're careful to put the BM down the toilet and wash our hands after wiping before they touch anything else. Everything stays cleaner that way.

Why do I have to go in the bathroom? I like to do it better outside.

If I let you do that, and if everyone else went outside too, pretty soon there would be germs all over. We wouldn't have clean places to walk on and it wouldn't smell nice, either. We have to take care that we flush our BM germs down the toilet, so they don't make other people sick.

Why do I have to wash my hands before I play with myself? Is it dirty down there?

No, it gets clean like the rest of you when you have a bath. But your hands might not be clean. Remember that we try to keep our hands clean by washing them often.

Why do I have to put clothes on?

You don't have to here at home, if it's warm enough. You *do* have to when company comes or when you are outside. The reason is, almost everybody likes it better for other people, who are not family, to be dressed. At home, they can decide what they want to do, just the way we decide for us here.

But if company comes, I'm *at home.*

That's true, but *they* have to wear clothes to get here, so *we* do too. People feel more comfortable when they're visiting if everybody wears clothes.

3

Threes and Fours

The two years between the third and fifth birthdays are often called the years of magic. Although the child's ability to think logically is growing, there are times when he or she will explain something in magical terms. There may be an imaginary playmate for solitary play. A boy may be convinced that when he grows up he'll marry his mother, or a girl her father.

Whatever the magic, it is important not to make fun of it or to scold or demean the child. Just give a simple explanation of the facts: "That's a good story, and it makes me happy that you like me so much you want to marry me, but fathers and mothers don't marry their children. When you are grown up you will find someone around your own age to marry. That way you will have your own new family and you will still be part of our old family, and our two families can visit together."

You may want then to ask yourself what might be underlying the need for this "magical" explanation. Has a parent been absent on a "long" trip (three days seems very long at this age) or perhaps working at the office past the children's bedtimes, or even perhaps cutting back too suddenly and prematurely on warmth, touching and cuddling, as mentioned in the last chapter? As the child grows and matures, parents and other adults inevitably take care of him or her differently, in ways they consider more appropriate to the new level of development. The child, however, is always of two minds about these changes, wanting to be "a big girl" or boy, but also to keep the privileges of babyhood. The conflict may be especially poignant if a new sibling is born in the family.

Children are often baffled by this conflict and by their continued yearning for intimate care from one or the other parent. Standards of behavior appropriate for a three-year-old, and parental pre-occupation with work, office, travel and the like, are difficult for the child to base in everyday reality. So the magical thinking follows: "When you are married you have special times with the person you love"; or "You get to stay up late"; or "She [or he] hugs you the most." Therefore, "We'll get married when I grow up and then everything will be okay."

You may want to consider how closely this kind of moral reasoning parallels that of teenagers when they say, "As soon as I have intercourse I'll be grown up," or "I need someone to love me because my [father, mother] doesn't, so I'll have a baby who will love me."

Such magical thinking is appropriate for a three-to-four-year-old who can't act on it and who can be given plenty of chances to grow toward more rational and moral reasoning. It is inappropriate and a danger signal when an eight-to-eleven-year-old is still reasoning at this low level. It is certainly so for a teenager. You will want to make corrections in reasoning for the three- and four-year-olds, but do it gently and patiently. You will be able to firm it all up in the coming "reality" years, beginning at five and six. Developing the capacity for making decisions on the basis of knowledge and reason is the foundation for morality.

At three and four, a child's sexuality is developing with the rest of his or her body. By the time the child is three, he or she has learned to define the physical boundaries between what is "me" and what is "someone else." Now it is the boundaries of behavior that the child must learn to understand; but sexuality in its broad, social aspects is difficult for a three- or four-year-old child to grasp. Specific sexual acts are generally hidden and the subject is not discussed the way other common parts of life are. There is plenty of room for confusion about why, for instance, it is okay to wear a skimpy swimsuit (publicly sexual) but not underwear (privately sexual). How and when does the child come to understand the subtleties of such differences?

The fact that excretory and reproductive functioning happen in the same small area of the body can be confusing for the three- and four-year-old. Experimenting with different ways to urinate fascinates some three-year-olds, especially girls, who often try to accomplish it standing up. Four-year-olds also want to know where babies come from and how they get out of the mother.

At this age children are very matter-of-fact about discussing how babies are made, but they are very concerned with elimination. They are keenly sensitive to parental attitudes about urine and feces that seem to carry an unpleasant connotation. They are very interested in what other people do in the bathroom and in verbal play: "You're a poo-poo!" "You're another poo-poo!" In upsetting situations children may clutch their genitals and feel a need to urinate.

Children will inevitably develop their own ideas about where babies come from regardless of what parents tell them. Even when they see adults having intercourse they seldom recognize that this is how babies are made. This is why the child may continue to ask the same questions over and over. He or she is simply trying to understand.

Because the capacity to handle the complexity of the reproductive process varies so widely among children of the same age, it is essential that parents keep listening to the child to help him or her sort through the magical confusions and illogical connections. This will have to happen a number of times, but each time can be an opportunity for providing not only facts, but attitudes, feelings, expectations and positive values. All this is part of the lives of all people all over the world.

Sex play between children of the same and opposite sexes goes on right through childhood without observable harm except when adults make an uproar about it. For children of three and four, handling their own genitals, cuddling, kissing and touching each other are common in both same-sex and other-sex play, with much tickling and giggling in between. All of this calls to mind the group play of puppies or kittens. By age four, sexual games such as "Doctor" and "Mommy and Daddy" are common and also very useful in realistically settling once and for all the question of genital differences between males and females.

It is interesting that, in spite of the undoubtable evidence that experiences of genital and bodily exploration and experimentation appear to be almost universal, many adults refuse to accept such behavior as natural in their children because they do not recall such sex play in their own childhood. You might try actively to probe your childhood experiences and see what you come up with. Bear in mind that "forgetting" most generally occurs because of the pain caused long ago by strong adult prohibitions, or by the frightening adult anger or punishment that may have accompanied the incidents.

Few parents are aware of how much a child's most lasting sex education is transmitted before nursery school. This education is based not so much on directly received information as on attitudes learned from parents, from other people and from television. Whether positive or negative, these sexual attitudes are being transmitted to the child, with or without words, in all kinds of ways.

The three-year-old is entering the peak period of language development, but parents are often afraid of the words that give young children straight factual information for fear of "putting ideas in their heads." But if the ideas were not already there, where would the questions come from? Like adults, children can only use information they can understand. Be concerned if you are explaining too little, not too much. You quickly will be able to tell whether the level of information you're giving is right.

Many parents worry unduly if a child has seen them making love. If parents stay calm and tell their children, "We are loving each other and playing sex games," the child will accept it and may even feel more comfortable about his or her own sexual activity.

Some parents even try to hide everyday affectionate demonstrativeness. This can indicate a wide range of sexual negatives and hang-ups that can weigh heavily on the lives of their children over the passage of time. Children delight in and thrive on love openly expressed among the people around them.

Obviously, avoiding a subject can often serve to draw attention to it. Without ignoring or evading a child's questions or feelings, however, there are also times to say simply: "That's the way we want it here in our house." Children who have confidence and trust in their parents' love for them, and in their willingness to answer all questions, will generally accept such decisions peacefully even though they might not understand or agree with them at the moment.

The child should leave these "magic" years with a sturdy sense of the realities of daily life, of who and what he or she is, and of Dad's and Mom's approval—even though parents will continue to push the child toward increasingly mature behavior.

Some parents are afraid to be open with their children about sex lest the youngsters share what they know with their playmates— whose parents may object. Children *always* share sexual information, whether you want them to or not. Despite that, what is important is that your child be able to depend on you always to tell him or her the truth. This will protect the child from potential harm, as well as from possible sexual dysfunction later in life, both of which have resulted many times from the untruths and myths passed around by children and even perpetuated by adults.

Don't shy away from opportunities that could provide openings for discussing sexuality or from raising questions about sex that your child may be longing to ask but afraid to bring up. In all the years to come, you'll want your child to be able to say to his or her friends with security and pride, "I'll ask Dad and Mom—they always tell me everything."

How come Daddy has nipples but he doesn't have breasts?

Men don't have breasts underneath their nipples because they don't breast-feed babies. Breasts are for mommies to feed their babies with, so mommies do.

Why is that breast bigger than this one?

Our whole bodies are built that way. Everybody has one foot a little bigger than the other, one leg a little longer or one breast a little bigger. It's different with different people.

How come your nipples are darker than Aunt May's?

Everybody is a little bit different from everybody else. You know some people are taller or fatter, with dark or light hair, or with big noses or smaller ones. Breasts and nipples and fingers and toes and all body parts are the same way.

What is a bellybutton for?

Nothing at all *now*. Before you were born, when you were growing inside me in a place called the uterus, the bellybutton was the place where a tube connected you and me. We call that tube the umbilical cord, and you got food through it until you were big enough to be born. The bellybutton shows the place where the umbilical cord used to be. After you were born, you didn't need it anymore.

What do you call this little bag under my penis? What is it for?

It is called the scrotum. It holds the two little round things that are called testes or balls. Those will make sperm when you are older, probably about thirteen. Men need sperm to do their part to make a new baby.

Why does skin hang down over the end of my penis but not over Tommy's?

That's because when you were born the doctor told us that leaving the skin on your penis was fine. It's called the foreskin, and Tommy's parents and doctor probably thought it should be taken off. When that's done it's called circumcision. Doctors and families have different ideas about this. Just remember to pull your foreskin back and wash your penis carefully every time you take a bath or shower.

Do girls ever get circumcised?

Almost never in this country. In some countries, they do circumcise girls, but we don't think that should ever be done.

Why do you have hair on your chest, Daddy?

That is one of the changes that can happen to some boys when they grow up and become men. It's a little bit different for each one. Some men have lots of body hair and some have only a little. Women also have body hair, but men almost always have more than women.

Will it hurt if I stick my finger in my vagina?

It won't hurt if you do it gently, but you shouldn't put any other things in that might scratch or might even poke a hole in it. Remember your vagina stretches slowly, so put your finger in carefully. And always wash your hands first.

Mommy, what's in that box under the sink, those white things?

I guess you mean my pads (tampons). It's what women wear to catch the flow that comes from the vagina for a few days every month. It's called menstruation. That's a really big word, so some people say "having your period." The flow is a reddish color because there is a little blood in it, and by wearing the pad (tampon), the stain won't get on my panties.

Do you have it?

Not right now, but I get it every month. All grown women do.

Does it hurt?

No, it isn't a hurt, it's just something that's natural.

Can you go to the bathroom then?

Yes, you can because it doesn't interfere with anything—you just remove the pad (tampon) when you go to the bathroom, wrap it up and throw it away. Then you put on a fresh one. (*For girls:* In a few years, maybe when you're around twelve, you'll be getting your period and then I'll show you all about it.)

Why do you get a period?

It's part of the way a woman's body gets ready to have a baby.

How do girls pee?

They usually sit down so they won't get their legs wet. A girl's peehole is inside her vulva. It doesn't stick out at the front like a boy's penis.

How can I stand up and pee like boys?

For girls: You can pee standing up if you spread your legs wide, right over the toilet, but if you get the seat wet you'll have to clean it up! Why don't you practice in the shower to see if you can do it without making a mess? It's really easier for women to sit down.

Why can't I sit down and relax when I urinate like you do?

For boys: You can if you feel like it, and some men like to. But you'll have to be careful to aim your penis straight down into the toilet bowl. If you get the seat or the floor wet, you'll have to clean it up!

Tommy said in real school the big kids in first grade have separate bathrooms for boys and girls. Why do they do that?

Because a lot of people feel that it's important for boys and girls to be separate when they go to the bathroom in a public place. When people are at home in their own family, they can make their own rules.

Why won't Grandpa let me hold the hose between my legs and squirt it?

I know it's fun. It's just that Grandpa gets upset when he thinks you are making jokes about things like peeing that he believes should be private. Try to remember that when he comes to visit. He's our guest when he is here, and we love him, so we should try not to upset him. When he isn't here you'll have lots of chances to play with the hose.

Why won't Laurie's mother let her and me go to the bathroom together when I'm playing over there?

She probably believes that boys and girls should be private from each other when they go to the bathroom, and that you're old enough now to understand that. She makes the rules at her house the way Daddy and I do here at our house.

Then why do we all go to the bathroom together at nursery school?

Maybe the nursery school teacher feels the way we do about bathrooms. If you want to be private about it, you can ask for privacy, but if you don't want to be private, then it's perfectly all right for everybody to go together.

Why doesn't Laurie have a penis? Was it cut off?

Of course not. No penis is cut off—you can be sure of that. Girls never have a penis. They have other things—a clitoris, for feeling good; a vagina, for making babies; and a urethra, to urinate. Boys do those things with their penis. If Laurie had a penis she would be a boy.

It isn't fair—Jimmy has a penis to play with and I don't. Why don't I? (See p. 25 for younger children.)

Because you are a girl. But think of all the nice things you have that Jimmy doesn't. Here, let's get a flashlight and a mirror and look. Remember to wash your hands first, though—often our hands are dirty with germs.

You notice how you have to spread the lips of your vulva in order to see inside? They help to keep everything protected and clean. You already know about this little button up here. It's your clitoris. It's specially for feeling good and it swells up when you play with it, just like Jimmy's penis. Here, right below your clitoris, is your urethra or peehole. Then your vagina is below that. They all feel good when you touch them. That's what girls have. Boys have penises.

Which is the right way to play with myself? Lisa just squeezes her legs together, but Sally puts her finger in her vagina.

You can try a lot of different ways—the right way is the one that feels best to you.

Daddy, which is the right way to play with myself?

Do it any way that feels good to you. There isn't any right way!

Janie says she has a vulva with lots of things in it and I can't have one. What's a vulva? Why can't I have one?

Because you are a boy. Girls and women have vulvas between their legs instead of a penis, as you and Daddy have. Inside the vulva they have a clitoris for touching and feeling good, and a urethra for urinating and a vagina opening for making a baby when they are grown. Boys don't have a vulva, but girls don't have a penis. Everybody gets to have something special.

What is a urethra?

That is the tube that connects the bladder with the outside of the body, either through the penis in men or, in women, to a place called the meatus (peehole), just below the clitoris inside the vulva.

Why does my penis get hard when I play with it?

You know how a hose feels stiff when water is running through it? Well, when you play with your penis to make it feel good, that makes extra blood run through it and that makes it get hard. The more you play with it, the better it feels and the harder it gets, until you feel satisfied. Then it gets soft again.

Why do I get wet between my legs when I play with myself?

Your body has a special way of making it feel even nicer when you're pleasuring yourself. It's called lubrication and is moisture that feels soft and slippery to the touch and keeps you from being too dry when you rub, just the way saliva does in your mouth.

Why is it all right for me to play with myself in my room but not in the living room?

Because most people think sex should be private. They get embarrassed if it's not, so we try not to do anything in front of them that could upset them. If you pleasure yourself in the living room while you're watching TV alone, that would be all right, but suppose someone came in to visit us and you forgot and kept on with it? That's why it's best to masturbate in a private place, like in your room, with the door closed so visitors would not come in unless you asked them to.

What is making love?

It is sharing the pleasure of yourself with someone else. It usually means sharing the pleasure of your body. You know how you make yourself feel good by touching your clitoris (penis). When you do that with another person—so you both feel good with each other —that's part of making love.

Who can make love?

People who are grown-up enough to know how to take good care of themselves and each other. Any two people who love and care for each other can make love.

Why did Jimmy say boys shouldn't kiss daddies on the mouth?

I don't know why he said it. Maybe in his family they don't kiss on the mouth, but you know you certainly can kiss *me* on the mouth, except when your mouth is full!

How come you make us keep our clothes on when we play?

I prefer that people wear clothes most of the time here in our house. Maybe that's because Grandma and Grandpa had it that way in their house when I was growing up. Each family can decide what the rules are going to be in their house, and maybe you will want to go without clothes in your own grown-up house. I just don't feel comfortable when we're naked with visitors around—whether they're children or grownups.

Jimmy's babysitter saw Jimmy and me with our clothes off and she said I was a bad girl and sent me home! Why did she do that?

You know how different families feel differently about the same things. Some people get upset even when little kids play sex games. We think those games are okay. So do you think you can remember to play them over *here*, and not to take your clothes off at Jimmy's house again? That would be a lot better.

Mom, if it's all right to see you in your swimsuit, why isn't it all right to see you in your underwear?

In our society, it's the custom that bathing suits are okay in public but underwear is not, even though they both cover about the same amount of skin. A lot of people see something sexual in underwear but not in bathing suits. I guess because of my own upbringing the only man I'm comfortable with in my bra and underpants is your father. It may be silly to think of underwear like that, but it's the way I feel.

Daddy, can I feel your penis?

No. Children and grownups shouldn't touch each other's genitals, like the penis or the vulva.

When you or Mommy bathe me and my sister, you touch our genitals. Why can't we?

That's different, and only for now, when we're teaching you how to bathe and keep yourselves clean. As soon as we feel you can do it the right way we won't have to bathe you anymore.

Is it bad when my sister and I touch each other in the bathtub?

No, that's two children together—a lot of brothers and sisters do that when they're little. As you get bigger you and your sister will probably find that each of you wants to bathe and get clean by yourself. By that time you'll probably have different ideas about whom you want to touch. For now, just remember it's not okay to play sex games with grownups and older children, even if they are in the family.

Do you and Daddy touch yourselves when you are in your room with the door closed?

Of course we do, and we also touch each other. There are lots of ways married people show they love each other, and that's one of them.

Why did you and Daddy close the door?

When Daddy and I want privacy we close the door. That means "Please stay out until we open it." When you want privacy in the bathroom or your bedroom just close the door and we won't come in either unless we knock first and you say, "Come in." If you say, "Please don't come in," we won't. We'd like you to do the same for us.

Do you love Daddy (Mommy) more than you love me?

No, of course not. You are my little girl (boy) and the love parents have for their children is very special. It's not the same as the love they have for their husband or wife, but it's just as important.

Daddy, why can't I sleep with you and Mommy? It's so cozy, I love it.

Well, in the first place we go to bed much later than you and we don't want to get up as early as you do. Secondly, you don't know it, but you roll and toss all over the bed when you're asleep—and your mother and I need our sleep. But last and most important, bed is your mother's and my very private place, where we can talk and joke and laugh and make love and sometimes even argue with each other. All that is private to *us*, just as *your* bed is private to *you*. So let's keep your bed visits for when we invite you on Sundays or special days—and not too early in the morning for those, either!

Where does the stork get babies from?

Who told you storks get babies?

The kids down the street.

Well, you and I know that's a funny, make-believe story. Don't you remember before your little brother (little sister, or a friend's baby) was born you put your hand on my (her) belly and felt him moving around inside? He was a real live baby then, and no stork brought him. I pushed him out through my vagina with my belly muscles and I held him in my arms the minute he was born, just the way I did with you.

How do you make babies?

The mother and father get together to make a baby. He puts his penis in her vagina so the sperm can go from his penis to join her egg. That's how a baby starts. (See p. 64 for older children.)

Why can't daddies have babies?

Only a woman has a special place in her body called a uterus for the baby to grow in. But making a baby takes both a mother *and* a father. A sperm from the father joins up with an ovum or egg from the mother and that starts making a baby.

Can children have babies? How old do you have to be? (See p. 65 for older children.)

When they get to be about thirteen or fourteen, girls and boys have bodies that can make babies. But this is really much too young to be prepared to have a baby. If it happens, it is sad for the girl and boy and it is sad for the baby, because its parents aren't nearly grown up enough to take care of it properly. Both of you should be finished with school and ready to work at a regular job. It's complicated to be a careful mother or father and take loving care of a baby.

How long does it take to make a baby?

The baby has to grow inside the mother for about nine months before it is big enough to be born.

How do you decide to have a girl baby or a boy baby?

You don't decide that. Nobody knows how to be sure that the baby will turn out to be one or the other. Anyhow, most people don't care about that as much as they care about having a healthy baby. So parents usually pick names for both kinds ahead of time, and love their baby whether it turns out to be a girl or a boy.

Can a woman have a baby without being married?

Yes, she can, but usually it's better for both mother and baby if they have a father living with them. But you know how Susie and her mother don't have a father living with them, and they love each other very much and take good care of each other. Fathers too can bring up their babies on their own if the mothers aren't living with them.

Can two men or two women have a baby?

No, only a man and a woman can make a baby together. It takes both his sperm and her egg, or ovum, together to do it. But two men or two women can be parents, if they decide to adopt a child or if they already have a child when they decide to live together and make a family.

Can I drink milk from your breasts like my baby brother does?

You can taste it if you want to. But I think you'll find that what tastes good to the baby doesn't seem as good to you now as it used to. You're a big girl (boy), and can eat many different kinds of food that your little brother can't eat yet. Even if it tasted good to you it wouldn't be enough food for you anyhow now that you're so big and have teeth to chew with. And your brother can't eat all the food you do, so he really needs the milk to get a good start in life.

If breasts are to feed a baby, why are you giving a bottle to my little brother?

Remember that I fed him at my breast for quite a long time? Now I need to get back to my job and I won't be around to feed him his lunch. He's a pretty big boy now and can drink cow's milk. This way the babysitter or your father, if he's home, can give it to him at lunch when I'm away, and I'll breast-feed him the other times.

or

Some mothers do nurse their babies and some decide not to. We give the baby his food from a bottle, but we make sure to snuggle him while we're doing it so that he'll know that we love him.

Why don't I have milk in my breasts like Mommy?

For girls: Because you are not grown up yet, and don't have a baby to feed. Even grown women with big breasts don't usually have milk unless they have recently had a baby that needs it.

For boys: Men and women are different and men have very small breasts. But usually only women who have babies can have milk in their breasts.

If you bottle-feed your baby, what happens to the milk in your breasts?

The breasts stop making milk when it isn't used.

4

Fives and Sixes

Children at five seem much more serious and self-assured than they were at four. They go to "real" school and feel they are thereby entering the "real" world. They understand their own limits, so they try first the things they feel they can do. Then they begin to measure themselves against the "big" children in first and second grades, wondering if they'll ever get there themselves. They love to copy adults as an important kind of rehearsal for the future. Observing this, adults should remember that children's play is not only play, but serious business as well. Sexual play is part of this serious business, and playing at adult relationships is an important trial experience for children.

Five-year-olds are clearly achievement-oriented: "What can you do that I don't know how to? What can I do that you can't?" They are now familiar enough with the physical differences between boys and girls, and comfortable enough with their competence in the bathroom to have lost their interest in what others do there. Interest in adult concerns and acting them out, especially those involving child care, are quite important, because the five-year-old is still unsure about the reasons for many adult activities, particularly those of the father, who is so often away from home.

Children of this age still have fanciful ideas about the baby-making process, and because delivery generally takes place in hospitals there is much confusion about just what happens there. Some children are under the impression that mothers buy babies, or that the baby must be cut out of the mother, since people go to hospitals for surgery. Some children still do not connect how a pregnant woman looks *outside* with a baby inside, especially if there have been no recent births in the family.

His or her own developing sexuality continues to be a central concern of every child. Though many people still believe in what Freud called the "latency" period (as a time when the child is relatively disinterested in sex), most leading child psychiatrists tell us that there is no such period. What happens is that because most children learn that sex is a parental no-no, they protect it for themselves by "going underground." Of course, they keep right on sharing with one another all the information (and misinformation) they may have about this powerful interest. This is *the* time to bring up sexual topics deliberately in order to encourage openness about sex for all members of the family. This can be done at the same time we emphasize family privacy about sexual matters with regard to the world outside.

School provides not only a new and possibly conflicting adult role model—the teacher—but also daily contacts with children from families with differing ideas about many aspects of life, including sex. The result may be conflicts in both attitudes and behavior. Until now most of the child's sexual experiences have been alone. Now such experiences expand to include other children, at school and in the neighborhood games which children use to explore sex together. Most of us remember "playing doctor" from our own childhood. Children play the game when they are three and four and continue to do so at five and six. It was and remains an all-time favorite. Some parents, forgetting their own childhood, make a fear- and guilt-ridden thing of this practically universal activity. There is little or no evidence that childhood sexual experiences with peers seriously damage later development and adjustment—as long as parents remain unruffled and deal comfortably though realistically with them without inflicting anger, punishment or guilt. As long as children are not exploited by other children or by adults, as long as the child wants to play and there is no coercion involved, most of these games do not harm. Instead, they help children learn what they have to know about their own bodies and about the bodies of others.

Thinking and talking about it together, parents can come to recognize that their child's private times with others of the same age, the casual, natural occasions with brothers and sisters, cousins and friends, can be accepted. In fact, rejoice when it happens in your own home, because then you can not only have some awareness of what is going on, but you can follow it up with calm discussion, making clear that it is truly okay to want to see how children of the same and opposite sex are made, and also making clear the limits and values that you wish to set in your family. Your assurance to them that their curiosity is reasonable and good reinforces your children's sureness that their bodies are just the way they ought to be. As early as possible children need to be very clear that sexual pleasure, intercourse and reproduction, while related to each other, are also experiences that can be separated one from the other. It is also important that they begin to understand the concepts of personal responsibility for the welfare of their own bodies as well as for the welfare of any other person with whom they have a sexual relationship. Although this is a time when a child can be at risk of becoming involved sexually with an older person, if there is a full understanding of what sex is all about, the child is less likely to be tricked or misled into an undesirable sexual encounter.

The drive for sexual pleasure never goes away. Many people remember beginning masturbation at about this time. The fives and sixes should be strengthening a capacity for sexual pleasure that can then extend smoothly into adult life. If your child doesn't masturbate, consider whether there may be negative feelings about the genitals. If so, try to make a special point of how the penis or the clitoris are natural parts of the body and that the pleasure they can give is good.

Much sexual socialization takes place without words. The five-year-old is very adept at reading body language. The way parents react to scenes on television, the tone of voice in overheard conversations about sexual topics, the tone of voice or facial expression in an unexpected sexual situation as well as the significant silences, the topics not discussed if the child is thought to be in hearing distance, all contribute to his or her sex education.

This also has the effect of making sex much more interesting, because it is treated as something so special. Though it may make the subject scary to the child, it is also likely to result in redoubled efforts to find out more about sex. You can be sure that children of this age have erotic interests. Too many parents have buried this knowledge from their own childhoods, and thus force their children to go to other children (and sometimes other adults) for reassurance instead of turning to their own parents.

Despite common agreement in our society that parents should be the ones to give their children sexual information, very few parents ever do so. Some mothers tell daughters about periods and pregnancy but boys almost never are told about these, nor are they even prepared for the ejaculation or wet dreams they should expect, the VD they should avoid, the contraception they should use, the rape they should shun or the tenderness and gentleness they should cultivate. Fathers give almost no sex information at all, even though ideally the male viewpoint is needed as a balance for both sons and daughters.

Traditionally, parents have had different standards for appropriate behavior for boys and girls. Boys have been rewarded for being assertive, impulsive, curious, exploring and taking leadership roles. Girls have been rewarded for being compliant, obedient, nurturing, empathic and concerned with group welfare. Even now—although our general attitude about these matters is changing—we can find ourselves going along, out of habit, with the traditional view that separates one kind of behavior and one set of values as proper for boys, and a very different kind of behavior and values as proper for girls. It always takes some time for the way we act to catch up with the way we think and feel. Most of us would prefer that our sons learn to be empathic, nurturing and concerned with group welfare, just as we would prefer that our daughters learn to be leaders and to be curious and assertive.

Traditional standards for boys and girls contribute to different attitudes about sexuality, and different kinds of sexual behavior in males as compared to females. If we expect and urge boys to see themselves as powerful, aggressive, ambitious and in control, we instruct them about one kind of sexual behavior. And if we expect and urge girls to be compliant and nurturing, obedient and passive, they are inclined to behave very differently as they act out their own sexual feelings and respond to the sexual advances of others. In other words, having different expectations for girls and boys because they are female and male results in damage to both, not only within themselves, but in their relationship to each other.

Boys tend to regard sexual experiences with others as exciting adventures that satisfy their curiosity; girls regard these same sexual encounters as invasive of privacy and demeaning, unless they are convinced that they are in love. Likewise, if the girl is approached by an adult she is likely to be more vulnerable than a boy because we have trained her to be more compliant and obedient.

The different expectations we have of boys and girls, and the way we train them, also directly affect how they will function sexually as adults. Passive women, women who are too "nice" to enjoy their sexuality, men who are aggressive or overly concerned with "performance" in bed or who rape, partners who never discuss their needs: these are some of the results of the sex roles we enforce on our growing girls and boys.

Parents are often upset when their children bring home from kindergarten and first grade the "dirty" words they've learned and use among themselves. Often they do not even know their exact meanings. It is up to the parents to help their children make the connections with the formal terms they should have learned earlier. When the child uses a term like "prick," for example, he or she should be told the word is slang for penis. A much better technique than punishment is for parents to let their children in on the well-kept sexual "secret," that many people use those same "dirty" words in private, even though it is not polite to do so in public. Laughing together at some of the ludicrous inconsistencies of the adult world breaks down barriers for both children and parents.

It is important that children understand that much sexual slang is derogatory to women. Parents have a real opportunity—we would even label it an obligation—to help their children understand the sexual exploitation of themselves and others implicit in a lot of sexual slang. How does a woman feel when her vagina is called a gash? And why should you call someone a prick? It just means penis, and a penis is something nice. Why use its nickname as an insult? This sort of slang is more often used in a manner that demeans girls and women, and in that way it reflects the same attitudes that underlie the predominance of rapes of women by men. Similarly, most sexual abuse of girl children involves little girls and adult men.

There is one inconsistency in our sexual vocabulary that has serious implications: Because for centuries women were not supposed to enjoy sex, the female sexual vocabulary is almost nonexistent. Though males currently use the Anglo-Saxon names for sexual parts and functions (cock/penis, cum/ejaculate, hard-on/erection and the like), equivalent terms for female parts and functions—for hardening of the clitoris, lubrication, the Grafenberg spot and orgasm, for instance—are not so commonly known.

It usually is not possible for an observer to see the girl's vagina become lubricated, or her clitoris hardening inside her vulva, so no one knows when she is aroused unless she tells them. Since she has no words for telling, she herself may even fail to recognize these signs as sexual. A male erection is easy to see, but without a similar nonverbal way of communicating arousal, the girl is not even sure of her sensations and feelings, much less able to express them.

There is lot of evidence that children act responsibly when they are provided with reasonable models. Parents can reinforce their own basic moral and value systems by being open to helping the child process new ideas picked up at school and from peers. For example, every week or so at the dinner table parents can play a running game of "What kinds of funny (or different or crazy) sex ideas did the kids talk about *this* week?" By such encouraging conversations, parents can continuously reinforce that they are available as resources for their children's sexual growth. The casually offered information that insertion of some object other than a finger into any orifice might be dangerous, the suggestions that there exists more than one way to masturbate or have intercourse or make love, can be dropped into a conversation. These comments serve to reinforce the child's growing sense that "I own and am therefore responsible for my body and its pleasures and its actions, and I can safely share my sex questions and feelings with my parents."

"It's six o'clock—did you hug your child today?" is a public relations message to parents that hugging and cuddling and touching are ways to nurture a child. Children and adults never lose the need for skin contact because it brings back the warmth and security we knew as infants. But mothers and fathers who understand this about each other may be afraid of the feelings that touching may arouse in their children—and in themselves. If such feelings occur, whether in parent or child, they can and should be brought out into the open and freely discussed as normal. They are not cause for alarm but opportunities to talk about what sexual responses and what reactions are appropriate with whom.

It can be illuminating and comforting for a child to learn that the good sexual feelings he or she experiences are the same as Mommy and Daddy have, and relate to why they love each other. Then discussion of the inappropriateness of acting sexually on such feelings when they are between parents and children will help the child accept responsibility for control of his or her own sexuality. Every person, whether a child or an adult, *always* has the option of saying "no" to any sexual advance. It is essential to emphasize that *both* people involved must feel comfortable with what is happening. Sex will not be pleasurable if either one is not comfortable with the partner, who must be an appropriate one, a person of approximately equal power. The inappropriateness of sex between adults and children, or teenagers and children (one who is much more powerful and one who is much less powerful) should always be talked about, not kept hidden. Child molestation must be understood to be avoided.

Here again, the sexual explorations of children with others in the same age group can be a safety factor. If your child has well-adjusted friends *of his or her own age*, you can be sure that occasional sex games will be more than balanced by all sorts of other kinds of games and by the mutual supportiveness and protectiveness of the group's feelings for one another. If you can welcome the children into your home for their play, you will have some sense of "where they are at," and can sense their evolution, not just as your child's playmates, but as people learning how to deal with each other socially—and sometimes sexually.

What is a period?

That's short for *menstrual* period. Most women menstruate about every twenty-eight days for a *period* of several days. A woman's uterus gets ready every month to grow a baby by developing a lining from blood and other fluids to make it comfortable. If no baby has been started during the month, this lining fluid flows out of the woman's body. That's called menstruating, or a period.

I saw Sis take something out from between her legs and it was all bloody. Is she hurt? What was that thing?

No, your sister is not hurt. She is having her period. She's menstruating. What you saw was probably a tampon or sanitary napkin. It's like a piece of soft cotton that's used to catch the blood and fluid that comes from every woman's vagina once a month. Here, I'll show you one that hasn't been used.

Why is my penis so small?

Your penis is just the right size for you when you are your age. When you are a teenager it will grow much bigger and get to be grown-up size.

Would it hurt me if pee gets into my vagina?

No, it wouldn't—urine is perfectly clean.

Why can't I pee when my penis is hard?

A hard penis is for pleasuring and a soft penis is for peeing. It's made that way on purpose, so both things can't happen at the same time. If it wasn't that way, you might do one thing when you meant to do the other.

Why am I supposed to wipe from front to back?

Urine is clean, but your bowel movement contains tiny things called germs. Once they come out from your body in a bowel movement they could cause an infection if they got into the wrong place, like your peehole (urethra) or your vagina. That's why you should always remember to wipe from front to back, even if you only urinated, and also to wash your hands afterwards. (See p. 28 for younger children.)

How big was I when my penis fell off? I can't remember!

It never did because you never ever had one. Girls don't have penises—only boys do. Boys never have clitorises—only girls do. That's how you can tell who is a boy and who is a girl when they are born and ever after.

Why does my penis get hard?

Because when you play with it to feel good, more blood flows into it. That makes it get hard. That's the way it's meant to be. When your penis is hard, that's called having an erection. Girls' clitorises get hard the same way when they play with them.

What makes my clitoris get hard?

When you play with it to feel good, more blood flows into it. That makes it hard. That's the way it's made to be. Boys' penises get hard the same way.

If a stiff penis bends, is something wrong with it?

Definitely not. Most stiff penises do bend, some up, some to left or right, and a few down. Some stick straight out. They're all perfectly normal.

If a boy's penis gets hard when he plays with it, what happens to a girl when she plays with herself?

Her sex organs swell up, too. The clitoris stiffens and the inner lips of the vulva become swollen with blood just like your penis does.

What is an orgasm? (What is a climax?)

When a person is masturbating, or being touched and loved by another person, they can reach a point of the most excitement and pleasure that is called an orgasm or, in slang, coming. They might tremble with pleasure, or shout out, or their bodies might get flushed or stiff. An orgasm feels wonderful. Climax is another word that means the same as orgasm. (See p. 40 for younger children.)

Why does my body feel funny and my bottom jerk after I've rubbed my clitoris (penis) for a while?

Because when you play with it long enough to feel really good the muscles around your genitals get excited. Then something pleasurable happens that we call an orgasm, or a climax. Your inside muscles contract several times and that makes your bottom jerk.

Is there something wrong with me if I don't want to masturbate?

No, of course not. People masturbate sometimes in their life and other times they don't. Some people hardly ever masturbate. Others do it several times a day. Both are perfectly okay. It's up to you.

Ann says she masturbates by sticking a pencil in her vagina. Doesn't that hurt?

It might hurt her, yes. Generally it's not a good idea to put anything except your own fingers into your vagina or other body openings.

What is a hard-on (erection)? Sally said Joey had a hard-on but she wouldn't tell me what she meant.

The right word is erection. It's when the penis gets hard when a man or boy is feeling sexual pleasure. Hard-on is a slang word for that, and we'd rather use the right word. Remember that if you use the slang, do it in private because many people might be upset by such language.

Joe said if Dad catches me masturbating he'll cut my penis off. Will he?

Of *course* not! No one ever cut a little boy's penis off. That's a very important part of you, just the way Dad's penis is an important part of him. And masturbation is a nice part of practically everybody's life.

Can the doctor or anybody else tell if I've been masturbating?

No, there's no way for anyone to know unless you want to tell them.

Jimmie and I were playing doctor. He said I should kiss his sore penis to make it well. Would it be okay, to do that?

Kissing is one of the ways we pleasure each other, when we know and trust each other very well. What did you do finally about Jimmie's sore penis? (See next question.)

I kissed Jimmie's penis after he kissed my vulva. Is that making love?

That's one kind of making love. Usually we save lovemaking for people who are very, very special to us. And it's not ever something that we *have* to do—only if we really want to be that close and trusting with the other person.

I woke up and heard you crying so I came in. Why was Daddy jumping on you and making you scream?

I wasn't crying, we were pleasuring each other. Grownups like to play together just the way kids do. Daddy and I love each other and so we were enjoying each other by having intercourse. I was making pleasure noises, not pain noises. Next time you'll know that's all it is if you wake up. Meanwhile, we'd like you to remember that whenever you see a closed door it means "Knock first," then wait until you are invited before coming in. Everybody likes privacy sometimes.

What is intercourse?

Intercourse, or sexual intercourse, takes place when a man's penis is inside a woman's vagina.

What's rape?

Rape is when a person uses fear or force or physical strength to make somebody have sex when he or she doesn't want to. It is a terrible thing to do to anyone. People who rape are almost always men.

Does rape hurt?

Yes, because one person is forcing the other. It not only hurts the body, it makes the man or woman being forced feel terrible, degraded and used. Sex is something both people should want. It should *never* be forced.

They told us at school to be extra careful to stay away from strangers in strange cars. Jimmie said that's because there's a sex fiend around who's been bothering kids. What does that mean?

It means a person who wants to do sexual things with children. You know how we've always warned you not to get in a stranger's car, and to be careful about strangers who seem extra friendly with kids when there's no grownup around? They may say they only want to play a game, but some of those strangers who appear to be just friendly are really disturbed. They want to have sex with little kids, or rape them or maybe hurt them in other ways, too. Sex between grownups and children is not right. Of course, sometimes these are just friendly people, but there's no way you could tell. I think that anyone who really wants to be nice to a kid should first meet the teacher or parent or some grownup the child trusts. The best thing is for all you kids to stay together and not wander off alone, especially not with strangers.

Daddy, how come it's all right for me to go without clothes at home when only our family is here, but you and Mommy don't?

Your mother and I feel more comfortable with clothes on most of the time. It isn't that we don't want you to see us without clothes— you know sometimes you see us when we are dressing—but most grownups are so much in the habit of wearing clothes all the time that they don't feel quite right without them. You'll probably find that as you get older you will want to wear them most of the time too. Some people, though, do like to go without clothes in their families. (See p. 28 for younger children.)

What about taking showers together? Lisa's parents let her shower with them.

That's another thing that each family decides is comfortable or not. I know your cousin Lisa takes showers with her parents, but remember her big brother and sister don't. Lots of people feel it is all right with children your age, but that when they are bigger they should shower alone. Each family makes its own decisions.

How come you and Daddy let me come into the bathroom when you shower but Tommy's mother won't let him?

Different families feel differently about bathroom-sharing. We don't mind if you come in while we shower, but we wouldn't want you to come in while we are on the toilet. Some families don't care about either one, and others don't like to share the bathroom at all any time. It all depends on what makes each family feel comfortable.

Why were the big kids laughing when Spot got on that other dog's back?

Spot and the other dog were having intercourse—sometimes called mating. That's how dogs make puppies. Sometimes children think it's funny to watch dogs having intercourse because people make sex such a big secret.

Could a dog and a person make a baby together?

No, humans can have babies only with other humans. And it would take a male dog and a female dog to make puppies.

Why do I have to wear panties all the time under my clothes?

Because your genitals are easily seen when you don't have your panties on under your dress, and it isn't considered proper to expose the genitals in public. If you want to go without panties in private, here at home, you may, but when you are visiting, keep your panties on.

Are pictures of naked people bad?

No, they aren't. We think they can be beautiful, especially when they're made by great artists. I have a book here, let's look at some together.

What does "fucking" mean?

It means having intercourse, when a man's penis is inside a woman's vagina. "Fuck" is a slang term that shouldn't be used in public. It is not polite and would be considered a bad word by many people, even though some may use it in private. So when you are with other people never say the word "fucking" aloud, no matter what others do. And here in our family please use it as little as possible.

What is a cunt?

"Cunt" is a slang word for vagina. There are several other words for vagina that are just as rude. I certainly wouldn't like to hear any woman's vagina referred to like that, though some people do use the word in private, without meaning it as an insult. Never use a slang word like that in public.

What does "whore" mean?

"Whore" is the slang term for someone who is a prostitute. That's a person who has intercourse for money and not for love. It's a word that is always used as an insult.

What does "prick" mean?

That is a slang word for penis. Other words you may hear are dong, peter, cock or shaft. Never use one of those slang words in public. It isn't polite and it upsets many people. What you say in private is up to you—many people use sex slang in private. Other people feel it's better to call things by their proper names.

Why did Sammy tell me his penis is bad? Is mine bad?
For girls: **Sally's mother said her vagina is nasty. Is mine?**

I don't know why anybody says that. Some people have different ways of thinking about things than we do. We don't believe a penis or a vulva *can* be bad. Yours certainly isn't; nobody's is.

If God made me, why did He make me bad between my legs? Did He make me wrong?

God didn't make you wrong. He made you right. You're not bad between your legs but good, otherwise how could all boy babies and girl babies—everybody ever born—hundreds and thousands and millions and billions, have been made that way?

How does the daddy's sperm get in the mommy?

A man's penis gets hard in erection. Then he puts it into the woman's vagina, where it ejaculates the sperm. When a man's penis is in a woman's vagina, that's called sexual intercourse. (See p. 65 for younger children.)

What does "ejaculate" mean?

That is when something called semen, that has the sperm in it, shoots out of a man's penis. It usually happens only when he has an orgasm.

JoAnn's mother said God put her baby brother inside her before he was born. How did God do that?

JoAnn's mother probably meant that she was thankful to God that she and her husband were to have another baby. But she and you and I all know that the real way a baby gets made is by intercourse between a man and a woman.

Have I got a seed in me?

No, you haven't, not a single one. Only plants have seeds. What you and all girls have is called an ovum, which means egg. It has no shell, but is like a very small bit of clear jelly, about the size of a dot. You were born with lots of these in your ovaries. They are still there, but they aren't ready yet to meet a sperm and start a baby.

Jimmie said his parents found him under a bush! Is Jimmie an orphan?

You don't think Jimmie really believes that, do you? Jimmie knows as well as you do that a baby is made by a mommy and daddy making love—having intercourse. That way the daddy's sperm can join the mommy's egg. Sometimes people say something like that about a bush because they think it's hard for children to understand about sex. *I* think maybe the bush story is harder to understand!

When is a boy old enough to make a baby?

When he's old enough to ejaculate. The time when he begins to be able to do that is called "puberty," somewhere around age thirteen. Some ejaculate a little sooner and some a little later, but all boys get there eventually. Of course, thirteen isn't nearly old enough to be a father and take good care of a baby! That's a big, important job that should wait until you've done all the things teenagers want to do. You may not be ready to take on the responsibility of being a father until you're in your twenties or thirties or forties. (See p. 45 for younger children.)

When is a girl old enough to make a baby?

There are two parts to your question. A girl's body is old enough to make a baby when she gets to look pretty much like a grown-up woman and her breasts grow and she has menstrual periods. That's usually some time when she is in junior high school, about as old as your babysitters. By then her eggs are ready to join with a sperm and her uterus or womb can make a nice soft lining for the baby to grow in.

But the other part of your question is about when a girl is old enough to be a mother. Every baby that's born has to have someone to take care of him or her, and mothers and fathers have to be pretty grown-up people to take good care—it's a big job. So a girl should wait until she's had a chance to do all the kid things and teenage things she wants to do, and is getting old enough to act like a loving and caring grownup with other people, before she has a baby—and that may be as old as twenty, or thirty, or even forty. (See p. 45 for younger children.)

Frankie said when we grow up we can get together and put his thing in me and then he'll pee and we can get a baby.

Frankie has things pretty mixed up. You know a man can't pee when his penis is erect. Anyway, it's sperm meeting the woman's egg that makes a baby, not urine.

Can a black person and a white person have a baby?

Yes. The color of the skin has nothing to do with it. A mother and a father can be of any race.

Where was I before I was born?

You waited to get born for nine months inside my belly. There is a special sack we call the uterus or the womb for babies to grow in. Inside the uterus you were connected to my arteries and veins, where my blood runs, so you could share food and water and air with me. I held you in there for nine months, which is as long as from Hanuka or Christmas until summer. That's when you grew from a tiny speck, too little to be seen, to a baby big enough to be born, like this (indicate twenty inches with your hands).

Cindy said her new baby is floating in a bag of water inside her belly. How come it doesn't drown in there?

Cindy is right. The baby *does* float in the water bag so it will stay warm and not get bumped. Drowning happens when someone breathes in water instead of the air we have to have to stay alive. The baby won't need to breathe the way we do until after it gets born, so it *can't* drown while it's still inside Cindy.

Do mommies have to have their bellies cut open to get the babies out?

No, most of the time they don't. Usually the baby comes out through the vagina. Once in a while a baby doesn't come out easily that way, so the doctor makes an opening in the belly and the uterus and takes it out. Then he sews everything together and it all heals up.

Do mommies have to go to the hospital to have babies?

Most mothers do go to the hospital, but some have their babies born at home.

Can people make babies if they aren't married?

Yes, they can, and sometimes they do. A baby can only be started when there is intercourse between a man and woman—whether they're married or not. Most people get married before they have babies because they believe that's the best way to live together as a family.

Mary Sue said good mommies and daddies have lots of children like her family has. Why don't you get a baby, so I can have a brother or sister to play with?

People can choose how many children to have. Some choose to have more than others, the way Mary Sue's mother and father did. We wanted to have only you because we feel that we can take care of one child better than we could take care of more than one.

5

Seven through Nine

The years between the seventh and tenth birthdays are crucial for today's parents, who must bring up their children in a world that not only differs from the one they grew up in, but that continues to change relentlessly. Between seven and ten, rising pressures of outside influences compete with those of parents. Teachers are important, the media are powerful, but the specific influence of the many hours spent with peers is strongest of all.

Peer groups stimulate and expand children's curiosity and interests as they continue to try to gain mastery of their world and of themselves. They go on being highly interested in sexual matters, despite Freud's suggestion that sex was not a major interest in these years. A great deal of research among the current generation of young people has shown Freud's theory doesn't apply—at least in the United States.

Seven-year-olds are sufficiently aware of adult standards to be very self-conscious about their failures, mistakes or fears. They are adept at hiding their sexual interests, and have so well internalized adult reactions to sex that they may go to great lengths to avoid nudity or being touched. At the same time they are continuing sex play, especially with same-sex peers. Since it's easier to talk to adults about pregnancy and birth, children are more likely to focus the sexual curiosity they admit to in this area. Girls continue to play house, while boys band together to assert their independence in secret clubs and the like.

Try to take a long, honest look backward to your own childhood. This can help you understand and accept that your children are bound to express themselves sexually throughout their developmental years. Learning how this sexual interest is expressed is important in order for it to be dealt with to everybody's advantage.

The sensitivities, self-consciousness and withdrawal from closeness in seven-year-olds can be striking. Sometimes these can reflect difficulties in adjustments at school or too heavy demands for achievement being made on a child. This can be especially hard on boys, for this is also a period when girls tend to be better than boys in reading.

At this age a boy's father may be overinsistent on "manly" behavior and may punch and play too boisterously. A doting father may try to keep his daughter the "pretty little doll" she has always seemed to him—just at the time she is becoming aware of herself as a sensitive and vulnerable sexual being. What both boys and girls need from parents at this point is more, not less, tenderness and touching. Like sponges, they will absorb all the undemanding support you can give them. They are *persons* who need your love and approval *just as they are* until they have worked out for themselves how they would like to be different.

Parents should be careful to soften the effect on children of TV, newspapers, magazines and movies. In contrast to our position—that children need to be lovingly taught facts and attitudes about their own sexuality, appropriately expressed, experienced and enjoyed—there are strong conventions in our society that refer to sex almost exclusively as a commodity. These are, at base, linked with the buying and selling of services and goods (like blue jeans) many of which have nothing intrinsically to do with sex. Sexual relations are not portrayed as expressions of love but as acts of seduction and exploitation between men and women. From the afternoon situation comedies to the dolls promoted to preteen girls, from the linking of sex and violence in TV shows and films to the ads seen virtually everywhere, our children are encouraged to imitate, at an early age, the media-created adults they see playing sexual games.

This public pandering of sex is correctly understood by children to be dangerous and somewhat illicit. Our sons feel challenged to imitate the sexually explicit postures of rock stars, and our daughters hide their youthful freshness behind heavy makeup. The danger is that they will not only be pulled into enacting the exploitative sexuality they see portrayed, but also that they will believe that sexuality can *only* be linked with violence, commercial exchanges and shallow relationships. This can keep them from understanding that sexuality can bring self-knowledge and genuinely caring and respectful relationships.

Censorship simply doesn't work: There are far too many opportunities for children to absorb these cultural attitudes. But as parents we can be alert to opportunities to open conversations about those attitudes that we are not comfortable with. Watch TV with your children. Invite discussion by asking, "What do you think that girl meant by walking the way she did past that group of men? What were they saying when they laughed and whistled at her?" Exchange opinions and interpretations with your children, and allow them to know that there is another way to understand sexuality besides the one they see in the media.

At about eight, children shift their interest from same-sex friends to those of the other sex. Girls tease boys or boys chase girls and many of these same children are also involved in boy-girl sex play, which may in some instances even include intercourse.

The shift toward cross-sex interest continues for nine-year-olds, who are becoming very conscious of the possible onset of puberty, teasing about boy or girl friends, and playing kissing games which, with no adults around, often go further. In some communities children of this age engage in group dating.

Most children know a good deal about pregnancy by the end of the ninth year, but far too few have ever heard about contraception. It should therefore come as no surprise that several thousand ten-year-old girls become pregnant every year, some before they have even menstruated. The number of ten-year-old boys who become fathers is unknown.

Children continue to have sexual fantasies, and thoughts about being sexual with a parent or someone of the same sex make some children extremely anxious. Parents will understand from similar feelings of their own how feared these fantasies can be. Try to make clear to your children this very reassuring fact: Fantasy of any kind, because it does not become true but remains fantasy, is a safe way to deal with one's curiosities and feelings about sex. Through such daydreams, it is possible to explore sexual activities or relationships that in reality we may not want to make come true, or that we know would not be appropriate.

In England and the United States there is fear of and a strong taboo against parent-child sexual interaction. This too often results in such a totally hands-off reaction by parents that it can seriously interfere with family intimacy. Fearing that touching, cuddling and other expressions of intimacy might lead to undesirable sexual feelings, some parents go so far as never to touch or show tender interest to their children—or even to each other in their presence. This can be especially devastating to the child who is approaching puberty, as are many nine- and ten-year-olds.

Many people abruptly cut off expressions of physical affection or discussions of sex because they are afraid erotic feelings might be aroused among family members. The best and healthiest way for parents and children both is simply and openly to acknowledge these feelings. When you put them into words (see pp. 9–11) the child is reassured that such ideas are common. Then, make it clear that there is nothing to be afraid of, because having the feeling doesn't mean you have to act on it. Openly discuss with the children how inappropriate it would be to let such feelings lead you into sexual activity together. This will give you all a feeling of family strength, and the recognition that each one of you is competent to manage your own sexuality in responsible and wise ways. This preserves intact the mutual bonds of intimacy between parents and children, and makes possible the continued warm flow of expressions of affection among you. At the same time, it gives you the chance to warn children about sexual exploitation by adults. As you make clear how healthy and caring people manage their sexual needs and desires, you can explain that nobody should feel coerced or coerce others into doing things they don't want to do.

Children usually learn a good deal about sex from same-sex playmates. A boy finds out how his body works, and how he might act, from other boys. Girls do the same with other girls. Although in many families the mother has been the parent who talked with the children about sex, answering their spontaneous questions when they were together in the house, most men can recall how much they learned about male sexuality from their peers—comparing erections, watching each other masturbate, handling each other's genitals, even experimenting with oral-genital and anal-genital sexual contact.

It seems that this sort of sexual play and sexual learning in the years from middle childhood through adolescence is more universally experienced, and more emphatically remembered, by boys than by girls. There are several reasons for this. First, what girls learn from their mothers about their own bodies is more extensive and more authentic than what boys usually learn from their parents, so boys, needing to learn somehow, do so by direct experience from *their* real authorities—other boys. Second, a boy's erect penis is more difficult to ignore (in the locker room, for example) than a girl's erect clitoris, which cannot be seen, and that makes for more opportunities for boys to explore, talk and play. Third, because of sex-role stereotyping, girls have—in the past—usually been given some message that sex was, for them, both dirty and dangerous; their peer-group experimentation was, therefore, often less fully expressed as well as more furtive. Finally, because sexual interest has been forbidden more to girls than to boys, it has been easier for girls to "forget" or suppress their childhood and adolescent sexual play and experimentation. Given an opportunity to remember, without censure, and to share personal history with other women, most do remember occasions of peer-group sexual learning. There is considerable likelihood that the girl's early same-sex experiences with sexual feelings and behavior will have been with only one other girl on each occasion, although girls do, also, learn about these things in groups, especially at "sleepovers," just as boys are likely to have not only group experience but also experiments with just one other boy.

Parents sometimes worry that this same-sex peer-group experimentation in the years of middle childhood and just before and during adolescence might lead to homosexual preference in later years. Researchers generally agree that they can find no single or even predominant cause for homosexual preference, and there is no evidence that early sexual experience with a child of the same sex is in any way a significant reason for an adult choice of homo-sexual life style. Same-sex experimentation is nearly universal, and most children who experience this kind of learning about themselves grow up to become adults who prefer heterosexual relationships.

In summary, in the matter of sex, what children need from parents at this stage of their life is:

· *Accurate, reliable information, offered without bias.* Good reading materials are plentiful today and can be left openly around the house for any and all family members to look at and talk about (see Reading List, p. 120).

· *Open discussions together about information, and about the parents' reactions to their children's questions.* Work at developing trust between you and your children. Try to adjust your relationship with your children to keep pace with their growth, which may be very rapid. If you are willing to share some of your own sexual thoughts and feelings, this may help your child be open with you. Once you have begun sharing facts, ideas and feelings at a level of trust that goes both ways, dialogue about sexuality—and other matters—can flourish in a way that you would never have believed possible.

· *Opinions when asked for*—rather than decisions or judgments, which tend to close off discussion too early.

· *Your own values expressed frankly in your own words* as the ones you truly believe in and try to live by. Young people almost always give these a lot of respect even when they don't share them.

· *Receptivity to your child's decisions* as they affect that child—who will then more easily accept your concern and interest in his or her welfare. This doesn't mean you will give up your responsi-bility to protect the child or to exercise judgment on what is good for him or her. It *does* mean you will not be arbitrary, but will make clear your respect for the child.

What does "puberty" mean?

Puberty is the time when the bodies of boys and girls change and develop toward manhood or womanhood. There is no exact time-table, because the process lasts over several years. People develop at very different rates: Normal girls might start at nine and others at sixteen; normal boys might start at ten and others at seventeen. Boys usually go through these changes later than girls.

At what age do boys start to shave?

That depends on the boy's individual timetable. Most do not begin to shave until seventeen or eighteen, but some start earlier.

Why does Aunt Alice have more pubic hair than you do?

Does she? Well, sometimes people in some families have more hair than in others—pubic hair, or hair on the head. Or maybe because my hair color is a little lighter, it just looks less than hers. But the important thing to remember is that the amount of hair or the size of breasts or any other measuring like that has nothing to do with having babies or sexual pleasure or any other parts of being a woman.

Dad, when I went to the gym with you and Uncle Bill the other day I saw how big your penises were. I'm scared mine will never get big enough.

My penis was like yours when I was your age, and so was Uncle Bill's. When you get to be a teenager—or maybe a little before that

—your penis will start to get big, too. And when you're a grownup it will be regular grown-up size.

Do girls have orgasms?

Absolutely. Like boys, girls can begin having them—or remember having them—at different ages. Your dad remembers one when he was around five. I remember an orgasm when I was quite a bit younger. Even small babies have orgasms—both girls and boys—although most parents aren't aware that they do.

I think I just had an orgasm like you told me about. Can boys have them too?

Yes, of course they can. Touching and loving feel just as good to boys and they get just as excited about it as girls do. Even baby boys, like baby girls, have orgasms.

Do a boy's and a girl's climax feel the same?

Nobody can say for sure because you can't ever be both a boy and a girl to check it out. But when either men or women have an orgasm the same kinds of things happen: Their pelvic muscles contract rhythmically—tighten up, then loosen, then tighten again. Nerve impulses set these contractions going in the same way for both males and females, so we might guess that the feelings are also very much the same. We may never really know for sure, just like we don't know for certain whether you see the color red the same way I do. Also, each of us experiences orgasms differently at different times.

We can also ask how you feel *about* the experience—good? bad? so-so? marvelous? nice? Probably there's no difference between men's and women's answers to that question. Some men and women feel one way, some feel another. It's a little like comparing how lemon pie tastes to you and to me—and even that can vary from time to time, as no two lemon pies that were made at different times could ever be judged to be exactly alike in taste.

What is that white stuff I saw coming out of my big brother's penis when he was masturbating?

That was semen. At puberty, around twelve or thirteen or older, a boy begins to ejaculate. What that means is that when he masturbates or has intercourse, semen, containing sperm, shoots out of his penis. That is called ejaculation. It happens when a man is most excited, having an orgasm or climax.

What is a sperm?

A sperm is a male sex cell. It carries half of the material from which any children he has will be made. The other half comes from the mother. The sperm is made in the testicles and a man has between 200,000 and 600,000 in each teaspoonful of semen that he ejaculates. You can imagine how tiny each one is! Each sperm has a tail to help it move up through the vagina, the cervix and the uterus to the Fallopian tube, where an ovum may be waiting to be fertilized.

Can a boy use up all his sperm if he has sex too much?

Absolutely not. Boys and men continue to make new sperm until the end of their lives.

Can you have sperm if you only have one testicle?

You certainly can, just as surely and as many as with two. Do you know someone with only one testicle? Sometimes one stays up in the body and only comes down to the scrotum during puberty.

Is it normal for one testicle to hang lower than the other?

It certainly is. If it did not, both testicles would be squeezed by the motion of the legs when a man or a boy walks.

When will my eggs be ready to make a baby?

First several things have to happen: You have to reach puberty. That usually happens when you're someplace between ten and fifteen years old. You begin to menstruate and your body changes: You get hair under your arms and pubic hair, your breasts and nipples grow and so does your vagina. All this happens because your ovaries are making a hormone called estrogen. Estrogen also helps your body grow to its full height and to change in shape to be like a woman, with rounded breasts and hips. At just about this time your ovaries begin to release eggs, one every month, so that you could become pregnant.

Can you get pregnant as soon as your eggs are ready?

No, it takes a lot more. If you have intercourse without using birth control, then you may get pregnant. The way it works is this: About eleven to fourteen days after you menstruate, one of your eggs ripens. It travels down a tube called the Fallopian tube. If a sperm comes up to meet it in the tube, the egg might be fertilized. Then it would go down the tube to the uterus to start becoming a baby. As soon as that happens, no more eggs will ripen until that baby is born.

Can you get a baby if a man puts his penis in your anus?

No, you can't, because there's no connection between the anus and the uterus. But if any of the semen should happen to drop even on the outside of the vulva, then a sperm might swim up through the vagina to where an ovum was, and *that* could start a baby. The way to keep from getting pregnant is to keep the sperm and the ovum apart at all times without missing *once*.

What's "the curse"?

A slang term for menstruation, like "monthlies," or period.

Will it hurt when I start my period?

No, you may not even realize you've started—the first time or two it may be just a brownish discharge. Have you noticed a yellowish discharge on your panties the past few months? That's normal, so you'll probably start to menstruate in the next six months. Carry a pad or tampon with you, just in case. And remember—it may look like blood, but when you have your period, there isn't actually that much blood; it's mostly body tissue.

Occasionally some girls and women feel cramping in their backs or pelvises when they menstruate. No one really knows why, but being tense or scared about it will just make it worse. Most of the time, though, having your period is no problem.

Why do some girls make such a big secret about menstruating?

That's an old-fashioned idea left over from their grandmothers and great-grandmothers, who thought that talking about things like getting pregnant was unladylike. Having menstrual periods is something that more than half the people in the world do every month for a large part of their lives. The best thing to do is just to deal with it as naturally as you do the other parts of your life.

How old will I be when I get hair on my genitals?

For girls: Hair growing on your genitals is one of the first changes of puberty. Puberty usually starts when you are a teenager, but it can start at an earlier age. Some girls, for instance, start the changes of puberty when they are nine or ten, and that's perfectly all right. With other girls it won't happen until they are as old as sixteen. That's okay too. You call tell this is so by looking at kids in the seventh, eighth and ninth grades—some are tall and look very grown up, and others are still short and look like young kids.

The body changes of puberty take three or four years to complete. Although they will not always happen in the same order, nevertheless, once they begin, these are the things you can look for:

First, your breasts swell slightly just under the nipples; sometimes they feel a little bit tender when this begins.

Second, your nipples and the area around the nipples (which we call the areola) grows bigger and darker.

Third, you get a few short hairs on the top of your vulva; we call these pubic hairs.

Fourth, you will grow much taller very fast, sometimes as much as two or three inches in less than a year!

Fifth, your pubic hair thickens, and there is some hair growing in your armpits.

Sixth, you start to have menstrual periods.

Seventh, your voice gets deeper, and you might have acne on your face or chest and back; your growth slows down, too.

After this period you will only grow another half-inch or so until your are seventeen or eighteen and your growth stops altogether.

For boys: In boys puberty can begin as early as ten or as late as eighteen or anywhere in between. It takes four or five years for all of the following changes to happen, although they will not always happen in this order:

First, your scrotum and testicles start to get bigger.

Second, there are a few short hairs growing above your penis; these are called pubic hairs.

Third, your penis gets longer and thicker.

Fourth, your voice starts to get deeper.

Fifth, you experience your first ejaculation, either voluntarily while you're awake or involuntarily in a wet dream.

Sixth, you will grow much taller very fast, sometimes as much as four or five inches in less than a year!

Seventh, your pubic hair thickens, and there is some hair growth in your armpits.

Eighth, your voice gets much deeper, and you might have acne on your face or chest and back; your growth slows down, too.

Ninth, hair begins growing on your upper lip and chin.

For both boys and girls: It is possible and normal to go through these changes in a slightly different order. All of these changes will happen to you, but we are each individuals and we each have our own special pattern and rate of growth.

How do boys masturbate?

Most boys stroke their penis up and down with their fingers or with their whole hand. Right under the head of the penis is a place which feels especially good because there are a lot of nerves there that give pleasure when touched. There are many other ways to do it, and each boy will usually try different things at different times to see which gives him the most pleasure.

How do girls masturbate?

Many different ways. A girl can do it by pressing her thighs together rhythmically. She can use her fingers or her hand to press against the whole vulva—her outside genitals—or to rub her clitoris. She can put a finger into her vagina and stroke in and out.

Some girls have noticed a place inside the vagina, right up behind the pubic bone, that feels very good to them when they stroke it. This place is called the Grafenberg spot or G-spot.

Will masturbation make my penis bigger (vulva or clitoris larger)?

Masturbation does not have any effect on the size or shape of sexual organs.

What exactly do you do when you make love?

"Making love" can include any or all the ways by which people can pleasure one another, such as cuddling, caressing, kissing, talking about sexual pleasure that they imagine, fondling, masturbating together, or touching each other's penis or clitoris and vagina or breasts or other parts of the body in many different ways—with hands, or mouths, or touching them together. When the penis touches inside the vagina, that's called intercourse.

The big kids were talking about "making out." What does that mean?

That's a slang word teenagers use for sex play. It can mean they are involved in almost any kind of touching and kissing but not having intercourse.

Why does getting married make babies come?

It isn't getting married that makes babies, it's having intercourse. When people are having intercourse to share pleasure, without wanting a baby, they use something called contraceptives. Contraceptives stop the man's sperm from getting to the woman's egg.

That way they can make love without starting a baby. When they *want* to have a baby, they have intercourse *without* using the contraceptives. Most people who decide to have a baby and want to make a family get married.

What does "contraceptive" mean?

It's a method to use so that you can have intercourse without getting pregnant. It's also called birth control. There are several kinds of contraception, and all of them are based on keeping the man's sperm and the woman's egg from getting together during intercourse or from attaching to the woman's uterus to start a pregnancy. We can talk about each one if you want to. They're called the diaphragm, condoms or rubbers, the Pill, the IUD and the cervical cap. (See details in Chapter 6, pp. 114–116.)

How often do married people have intercourse?

As often as they both wish. It is normal to have it three times a day or once a year or anything in between, depending on what the two partners want and what they work out with each other. It's important that they both *agree* on how often.

Do you automatically know how to have intercourse when you get married?

Not necessarily. If no one ever told either the man or the woman how to do it, they might figure it out by themselves or they might not. Intercourse is like any other skill, it has to be developed by practice and experimenting. Most people learn to do it in ways that please each other and themselves. When people love each other they want to learn how to give the other person pleasure.

What is VD? How do you get it?

Venereal disease, or VD, means a disease that is sexually transmitted, so now we call them STDs or *sexually transmitted diseases*.
These are infectious diseases that you cannot get from a toilet seat,
only through intimate sexual contact with another person who already has the disease. There are about sixty different kinds of
STDs known today. Some of them are serious, so everyone should
know about them and be careful not to get them.

If a woman with STD has a baby, will it hurt the baby?

Depending on what disease she has, it can. One kind is called
syphilis: If she has syphilis while she's pregnant, the baby could
be disfigured, mentally retarded, have a heart problem or be born
dead. If she has gonorrhea, which is a different kind of STD, the
baby could be blinded unless silver nitrate drops are put in its eyes
immediately after birth. The dangers are so real that a woman should
be examined or tested for sexually transmitted diseases as soon as
she becomes pregnant, and then should be retested during each
of the last three months of her pregnancy. Early treatment is most
important; it can protect the baby from being hurt.

When can I have intercourse?

When you care a lot for someone who cares a lot for you, and you
both trust and want the very best for each other and are ready to
be responsible for each other. For hundreds of years people in
many places around the world have said that intercourse should
happen only between two people who are married to each other—
not only in case a baby happens, but because most religious groups
believe this is the right way. Not everybody feels that way and
there is sometimes a difference between what people say they
should do and what they actually *do* do.

But even though we know this, these days you can find eleven-

and twelve-year-old girls having intercourse. Some of the girls are even getting pregnant. That certainly isn't responsible. We think you are intelligent and informed enough not to let this happen to you. You know there are ways other than intercourse of getting to know and relate to someone intimately. There are lots of ways for pleasuring each other. Intercourse should wait until you're grown up enough to take responsibility for contraception and possible pregnancy. We're very serious about this, so think carefully about it.

Do you and Daddy do it for fun?

Of course we do. We also did it to make a baby when we had you and your sister. We also have intercourse because we love each other very much and want to give each other pleasure.

Can two women make love?

Yes, by being tender with each other and by using their hands and mouths and clitorises and vaginas. Women who prefer to make love with other women are called lesbians, or gays or homosexuals.

Can two men make love?

Yes, by being tender with each other and by using their hands and mouths and penises and anuses. Men who prefer to make love with other men are called gays or homosexuals.

Why do some people think it's okay to kiss on the cheek but not on the mouth?

One reason is that little babies or very young children might catch germs through the mouth that could make them sick. But for older kids and adults usually cheek-kissing is for friendship and mouth-kissing for lovemaking and sex. Most people want to keep those two separate.

Mom, how come I can still take a shower with Dad but you don't like me to have one with you anymore?

It's not that I don't like it, it's that you're getting to be a man. In most families, mothers and almost-grown-up sons don't go naked together, or take showers together or have sex together. You're growing up, and soon you'll be ready to find people your own age to do those things with. But we sure are going to keep on loving each other and showing it. Come over here—I've got a hug to prove it.

Dad, I see you in swim trunks and I've seen you in the shower but you never let us see you in your jockey shorts. How come?

You're right. It's a funny situation. I guess it's because I was brought up to connect underwear with bedrooms and sex. I don't have any problem with your brother because he's a boy, but many people brought up the way I was keep feeling that sex is private and underwear is connected to sex, so underwear is private too! So no underwear in "public"—and that includes my own daughter! It may be silly, but it's the way I feel.

If a lot of people have intercourse because it feels good, why does anyone get married?

Most people don't get married just to have intercourse. They *can*, if they want to, have it without getting married. But many people still want to get married. It's one way you tell the world and each other that you belong together and want to be a family. Once they find someone they love and feel very special about, many people want to make that formal and legal by getting married, the way people have been doing for hundreds of years.

What does "fairy" ("dyke") mean?

That's an impolite slang term for homosexual. A homosexual, male *or* female, is someone who is really and truly turned on only by someone of his or her own sex. Another, better term for homosexual men is "gay." That is the word many homosexuals themselves like to use, and they call a heterosexual person "straight." Homosexual women usually prefer to be called lesbians. There's a lot to learn about homosexuality. It's too bad for everybody that so many people choose to remain ignorant about it.

Is it bad to be a homosexual?

We don't think so, but that's one of those questions that different people have different opinions about. Some people think that you should only have sexual relations with a person of the other sex, and that anybody who doesn't choose to do that is not doing the right thing. In this family we agree with the scientists and doctors who say that a homosexual is just different from a heterosexual, but not bad or sick or strange. Certain people who don't approve of homosexuals are sometimes very cruel to them, so many homosexuals are hurt and tend to be very private about their personal lives. That's too bad, we think, because it's very hard and sad to have to hide that you love someone.

If a boy dresses up in his mother's clothes is there something wrong with him?

Not necessarily. Most people are curious about the clothing of the other sex and try it on at some time or other. In our country girls are allowed to wear male clothing at any time, but when boys wear girls' clothes, people make fun of them. There's really nothing wrong with doing either one. Some grown men, including both heterosexuals and homosexuals, like to wear women's clothing from time to time. It can give them sexual pleasure. The slang term for this is "being in drag." Sometimes men dress up in women's clothes in order to make fun of women. This is a cruel, mocking kind of humor.

What does "P.G." mean?

That's slang for pregnant.

Will a blind (deaf, lame) person have a blind baby?

There are very few troubles, like being blind or deaf, that are passed from mother to baby. Specially trained people called genetic counselors can explain what the chances are of passing on the condition they have to a baby. Then people can decide whether it is okay for them to have their own baby or whether it is safer to adopt one.

What would make a deformed baby?

All babies are a little bit different from each other. Some babies are quite a bit different—a baby might be missing a hand, or not be able to see or have a big red mark on his or her skin. We're not always sure when we should think that the baby is "different" and when we should think it is "deformed." Sometimes in the past people thought that you were deformed if you had red hair. That's silly, isn't it? Anyway, it's usually kinder to talk about differences than to say "he's deformed!"

Some differences are inherited, which means that we are born with the same thing that our parent or grandparent has. Other problems happen when the mother is sick while she is pregnant, or doesn't have enough food, or takes dangerous drugs, or smokes or drinks alcohol.

What you have when you are born is called "congenital." Some congenital problems can be corrected—if your baby has a split upper lip, it can be sewn together. Some problems can't be corrected but they can be helped a lot—if the baby has very poor eyesight, then wearing strong glasses might help him see. And you know that people who are blind, or deaf, or missing part of an arm can live happy and useful lives.

We often don't understand *why* things like this happen to people, or to families, but we do understand that when we know someone with this kind of problem we learn a lot about courage and patience and being strong and loving.

What is a fetus?

We have to go backwards a little to answer that question. For the first eight weeks after the sperm meets the egg we call what's been created an embryo. After that, from eight weeks until it can stay alive after leaving the uterus depending on the size and development, it is called a fetus. After that it is a baby.

What is a cervix?

The cervix is an especially thick ring of powerful muscles that forms a passage from the uterus into the vagina. If you think of the uterus as a small upside-down pear, the cervix is at the bottom or "stem" end. If an egg is fertilized, the cervix clamps the opening between the vagina and the uterus closed and holds it shut for the nine months until the baby is ready to be born. Then, in a few hours, it stretches its opening large enough so that the baby's head and body can pass through it into the vagina and out into the world.

What is a uterus?

The uterus is an organ way down in the woman's pelvis, shaped something like a small upside-down pear. It is made of muscles, and is lined with soft, spongy glands that are full of blood. The menstrual flow comes from it each month, unless the woman is pregnant. When that happens, there is no more menstrual flow until after the baby is born. The uterus will grow along with the fetus—not just stretch, but develop more muscular tissue to make room for the growing fetus. Within six weeks after the child is born the uterus returns to its usual size.

What is the umbilical cord?

While the baby is in the uterus, a long tube called the umbilical cord connects its abdomen to the placenta. The cord contains veins and arteries that carry the baby's blood to and from the placenta in order that nourishment *for* the baby and waste products *from* the baby can be exchanged between the baby's blood and the mother's.

What is the placenta?

It is rather like a round sponge that grows inside the uterus until it is about the size of half a grapefruit. It is where veins and arteries come from the baby in the umbilical cord, and lie alongside the veins and arteries from the mother. These veins and arteries have very thin walls, and that's how nourishment from the mother's blood can seep or leak through into the baby's blood.

What does the baby eat inside the mother?

The mother's bloodstream carries nourishment for herself and also for her baby. It is transferred to the fetus's bloodstream through the thin walls of the blood vessels of the placenta. (See previous question.)

How does the fetus go to the bathroom in there?

There are no BMs, only urine, because the fetus isn't eating. In the placenta the urine from the fetus is transferred to the mother's bloodstream, which carries it away and discharges it with the mother's own urine.

What happens to the placenta after the baby is born?

It isn't needed anymore so it also gets born, a little while after the baby comes. It is called the afterbirth.

Does it hurt when the umbilical cord is cut?

No, there are no nerves in it, so it can't feel anything.

Can people make love when a baby is inside the woman?

Yes, there's plenty of room because the baby is inside the uterus. That's above the vagina, where the penis goes in. When she's very big in pregnancy it's more comfortable to make love if the woman is lying on her side.

Won't it hurt the baby?

No, the penis doesn't get anywhere near it.

Did you and Daddy have intercourse before I was born?

Yes, we surely did!

Was I there?

You certainly were—you were floating inside a sac of water, that was inside the uterus, which was inside me.

Did I see you do it?

No. Not only is it dark in there, but you were completely enclosed by the water bag in which you were floating and by the thick muscular wall of the uterus. You might have felt bouncing movements, and perhaps you could have heard some of the loving sounds of our voices, because sounds can get through. We think that some babies at birth may already be familiar with their own mother's voices because they've been hearing them. Anyway, isn't that a lovely thought?

What is incest?

Sexual intercourse between members of the same immediate family —father and daughter, mother and son—is called incest. No one believes incest is appropriate, and in almost every state it is against the law.

Even if they're in the same family, when an older person forces sex on a younger one, it's called rape. It's hard for children to refuse these kinds of advances, because older people have more power and children are used to doing what grownups ask them. We want you to understand and remember that your body is your own, and only you can say who may see or touch you. When you are uncomfortable about a situation, or when somebody's giving you a hard time and you are not sure what you should do, say a strong "no" and get help from another grownup.

What does "horny" mean?

It means that you feel sexually excited.

6

Ten through Twelve

Puberty is not a single happening, but a quite long procession of biologic changes. No matter at what age it begins, it still takes four to five years for boys and three to four years for girls to complete. The sequence of events leading to physiological and reproductive maturity is carefully detailed in Chapter 5 (pp. 43–93). We felt the information belonged there because of the great numbers of seven-to-nine-year-olds who ask, "When will I have my period?" or "When will I have my first ejaculation?" Knowing where they can look it up in this book can give your preteen children an understanding and a sense of being in charge of the whole self-engrossing business.

But these are just the facts. Children need to hear from you that, along with bodily maturation, you also expect that maturation will come in thoughts, feelings, attitudes and relationships. One way to assume and support your important role at this time is by thoroughly familiarizing yourself with the expected sequence of events.

Girls tend to begin the process a year and a half to two years earlier than boys, so it sometimes seems that they are ahead of boys their own age. But in a large group of same-grade boys and girls things eventually even out, and obviously everyone reaches puberty in the end. It is considered that puberty has been reached when the boy or girl achieves the capacity to reproduce. This is a very important time, when parents and children need to talk freely and often in order to understand everything thoroughly. And they can also rejoice together as the various stages make their appearance on the way to puberty.

Preparing children *for* puberty well ahead of its possible beginning is not difficult. Presumably they have already asked and learned something about it during the years before ten. If they continue to feel reassured that you are "askable," they will feel free to come immediately with any perplexing questions. Because talking takes away the strangeness and the fear, much of the worry will also go away. And parents can begin to think about the kind of ceremony they'd like to plan for the arrival of puberty in their children.

Reaching puberty is one of several important milestones in human life, and in many cultures there are "rites of passage" to mark this momentous event, to give public recognition to a private event. In the same fashion, when two people become engaged or married they are publicly proclaiming their private decision to become a couple and perhaps to have children together. Some families celebrate when their child reaches puberty by having a special dinner at a favorite restaurant or by breaking out a bottle of champagne. Jewish families have the bar or bas mitzvah. One way to celebrate might be some symbolic evidence that he or she, now able to make babies, is thus entering the world of adult responsibility. Some families offer their children the right to call their mother and father by their first names or to make some trip alone. Whatever symbol is chosen marks the recognition and confirmation that the child's body, with all of its functions, is good and important and acceptable to the most important people in the world—his or her family.

Because puberty changes in both boys and girls can begin as early as seven or as late as eighteen, one individual might literally still be a child by the twelfth birthday while another might be well into adolescence. However, half of all girls and almost that many boys reach puberty before thirteen.

The first signs of pubertal changes cause many parents to clamp down on physical expressions of affection or touching with their children. A child cannot help blaming this withdrawal specifically on the pubertal changes themselves, and may thus begin to hate them as "bad." Girls especially may have heard the menstrual period referred to as "the curse" and seen this "cursedness" confirmed by a parent's apparent withdrawal of affection. This can be devastating for some ten- or eleven-year-olds who may feel especially isolated.

If masturbation was interrupted at some previous time, it is often rediscovered now. Because their masturbation was thoroughly condemned in earlier years, some children have not since been able to enjoy self-pleasure. These children now get trapped in cycles of masturbation, guilt, futile struggles to abstain, more masturbation, more guilt, etc. You may remember such cycles from your own childhood as profoundly disturbing. If so, you'll want to help your child break them. Extra affection and reassurance coming from you that masturbation is permissible for everyone, will do it.

Erections come so easily and so often in boys just before puberty that by the time they're adolescent almost all boys can masturbate to ejaculation. Although fewer girls masturbate at this time, many do experience their first self-induced orgasm during these years.

Same-sex friendships continue to be a strong focus of sociability. Boys are most likely to learn about sex from other boys. Seeing who can pee further or who can ejaculate quickest may lead to masturbation while talking about girls, mutual masturbation, fellatio, acting out intercourse and anal intercourse. This kind of experimentation is generally not looked upon as homosexual by the boys themselves.

As with the younger groups, girls of this age are less likely than boys to engage in sex play in groups but they are somewhat more likely to exchange facts and techniques with one other girl and they do share "out-loud" sexual fantasies. Friendships with girls continue to be important throughout adolescence, and indeed through adult life as well.

Some other-sex friendships began at age ten or earlier and dating may also begin at this time. Children may feel ambivalent about beginning to play sex games with persons of the other sex. The changeover from "same-sex" to "other sex" in this play is made easier because preadolescents get the message from society that being a sex partner is the main prerequisite to being sexually mature. It therefore should come as no surprise that many of these preteens are having intercourse and, sometimes, mouth-genital contact, usually with partners their own age.

The years before puberty are the time children learn about their own sexuality. Interfering with that process can keep the child, when he or she reaches adolescence, from being able to focus on relating to others; the sexual focus is directed inward instead of outward. If the child is still preoccupied with getting in touch with his or her own sexuality, he or she will not be able to develop concern for another person, learn to plan and take responsibility for joint actions and become emotionally involved with others. The conflict could lead to a sexually exploitative relationship, involvement in a pregnancy or to sexual hurt of some kind for one or both involved.

These are the kinds of things that disturb what ought to be a smooth path into adolescence. It is distressing to realize that very few mothers and almost no fathers talk with their children about puberty, intercourse or premarital sex. Even fewer mention STDs (sexually transmitted diseases) or birth control.

Instead of this, sex usually has been discussed with children only in terms of reproduction. They have had no opportunity to learn about the closeness, intimacy and peaceful satisfaction that can arise out of loving, sexual union, for nobody ever talked to them about *feelings*. Children are often not aware that *the best part of marriage is not sex alone, but what it can mean within a loving, caring relationship.*

In each chapter of this book there have been some questions and answers that may seem to be beyond the interests or perhaps even the capabilities of the age group of that chapter. We did this deliberately, and do so again in this final chapter. There are always children in the upper limits of maturation who find themselves going through puberty at nine or ten years of age, while still in the fourth grade. The largest number, however, go through it at the seventh- and eighth-grade levels. Socially speaking, a few boys at nine or ten may be extremely self-conscious about their dark pubic hair, changing voices and enlarged penises. A few out of a group of same-age girls will already have pubic hair, breasts and menstrual periods. To look at these *sexually* mature boys and girls one would think that they belonged in the seventh or eighth grade; but no, they are correctly placed in the fourth or fifth grade according to their intellectual achievement and age levels. It is their social maturation levels that are at stake here.

If the parents have felt that they were "too young to be given sex information," then these children, having no explanation offered to them for their being "different," naturally are confused and may suffer keenly or else be misinformed about what is happening to them. So every once in a while, try to assess where your child is regarding his or her stage of sexual development. Consider whether or not the child has the sexual information needed to see him or her through that phase of development. A carefully thought out conversation can be casually opened something like this: "You know, you seem to have some of the signs of being on your way to puberty. That means you are going to mature early, the way some people do. That's perfectly normal and okay. We just have to make sure you're prepared. It looks as though you might expect your first ejaculation (menstrual period) some time in the next six or eight months. Do you feel all right about that? Would you like to ask me or your mother (father) some questions about it? Don't forget, we've both been through this too."

If whole families—including Grandma or Grandpa or other relatives—could get to feeling comfortable in just plain *talking* together about sex, not in hush-hush embarrassment but in the ordinary way one might talk about any subject of common interest, we firmly believe that there would be fewer runaways, or frantic teenagers seeking abortion, or too-young and ill-prepared parents abusing their children. Such talks *can* be free of embarrassment and as helpful as talks on any life-important subject.

In preparation, try backtracking in this book to check out what sexual areas you and your children might not yet have opened up. Before puberty hits is the time to catch up on things. When you spot a subject that you think ought at least to be touched on, you might bring it up by a variation of a technique mentioned earlier (see p. 53)—"So what crazy sex things did you kids talk about this week?" The variation for the older child is more direct: "We've been wondering if any of your friends ever bring up questions about things like exhibitionism (homosexuality, sex between family members). Lots of people worry about these needlessly, even adults do when they haven't had a chance to discuss them and learn the facts."

In the family that is open about discussing sexuality, it is fairly safe to take for granted that a youngster has sufficient information if he or she responds comfortably. But if you are more or less in the early stages of "opening up" with your child, don't take anything for granted. Pick a subject your child responds to when it is mentioned, and take it from there.

We urge that, during discussions, until total trust about sex is established among you, all adults agree to hold back on strong opinions or judgments. Masturbation, teen sex and homosexuality are probably the most difficult subjects for parents to remain neutral about. But try hard. Hang on to *facts*. Today almost all psychiatrists and other specialists agree on these three things:

1. Masturbation is an expected and valuable part of sexual life from our earliest to our last days. Its most important phase is in the early months and years of development, but it will never lose its significance and usefulness throughout life and into old age.

2. What we know for sure about homosexuality is that we don't know enough. There is little evidence that the family "does" anything to cause this sexual preference but, on the other hand, no one has made a convincing case for its being hereditary. Many experts feel that homosexuality develops before eight years of age. Others believe that people in our society are labeled too much, and that, without societal pressure to "decide" what you are, probably a lot of people would be closer to being bisexual; that is, they would have some homosexual experiences without being pushed to think that that made them "different" or that they had to have a special life style because of their sexual experiences. In fact, some people go through a homosexual "phase." Others are apparently bisexual, either for short periods or throughout their lives.

At present a small percent of the population is exclusively homosexual and remains that way throughout life. Therefore, homosexuals are everywhere. They work in all professions (medicine, law, theology, education), in sports (football, baseball, ice hockey, and tennis), in the arts, and in business and the trades. They are you and I, if we are heterosexual—except for their sexual orientation, and except for various problems *that come from the way they are treated by some heterosexuals.*

Homosexuality is not catching, like measles. Homosexuals very rarely rape or molest children. Such crimes are generally committed by heterosexuals. They feel exactly the same hunger and need for intimacy and touching and loving and being loved as do heterosexuals. The day one of your children informs you that he or she is gay, bear in mind that the child hasn't changed one bit from the day before you were told. *You* are the one who has changed: You now have a piece of information about your child that you didn't have twenty-four hours earlier—but *he or she is still the same child you have always loved.* How can your feelings toward him or her change?

Though they may have thought about it since childhood, adolescence is the time when many people confirm that they are homosexual. When you learn about this, the greatest gift to your child would be for you to accept it without hesitation, to put your arms around him or her, and to say, "I love you. Now, what can I do to be a good and supporting parent?"

3. Teenagers continue to be as interested in sex as they have been right along. For them, it is as natural and necessary as breathing to seek one or another kind of sexual expression. So concentrate on helping them: (a) to explore sexual life styles that might serve to increase their sense of self-mastery and good decision-making; (b) to explore and discover some of the many factors involved in friendships that are not sexual; (c) to think about when and how they might be tempted to take sexual advantage *of* someone, and the possible reasons for this; and (d) to identify when and how they could be taken sexual advantage of *by* someone, and the possible reasons for this.

The solution to the dilemma of the American child with respect to getting correct facts and developing good feelings about any and all aspects of sex, puberty and adolescence lies in the hands of parents. Schools can help only by complementing what parents do.

It is not yet too late for parents to move toward setting their children free from fear and anguish about something that is, after all, and quite simply, a gift of life itself.

This is a really tough time for me. Is there some way to grow up faster?

It may seem slow to you, but you are perfectly normal and one of millions and billions of girls and boys who have gone through puberty and lived! Talk to us whenever you feel like it about whatever comes up, either in your social life or in your sexual development.

My parents say when I get my first period they're going to take me out to dinner and celebrate. The other girls think this is weird, and that I shouldn't tell my parents when it happens. Is it weird?*

I'd say it's wonderful, not weird! Your father and mother want to celebrate something very important: Somebody they once knew as a small, helpless baby is suddenly becoming a woman. Their celebration on this important occasion can be called a *rite of passage*— a ceremony when you leave one phase of your life and enter the next one. Many people all over the world have these kinds of ceremonies. Your parents are proud of you and also proud of themselves for helping you to get along this well.

---

* Questions like this are sometimes asked of adults outside the family whom the child trusts.

Why do some girls get their periods at nine or ten and some not until sixteen?

Nobody knows for sure. Some think it could be due to heredity or geographic origins or racial backgrounds. It certainly can have something to do with the food you eat—children who don't eat good food may develop more slowly and menstruate or ejaculate later.

I've had pubic hair and breasts for a long time and I still don't have my period. Is something wrong?

It usually takes about eight months after your breasts develop. First you outgrew all your clothes, remember? Next your pubic hair will thicken, and *then* you'll have your first period.

How long does a period last?

After the first year of having menstrual periods, most women settle down to their own characteristic time periods. It could be three days or seven days, but the most usual is four to five days. The time between periods also varies, but mostly it's around twenty-eight days.

Now that I get my period, what if I skip a month? Does that mean I'm pregnant?

Not necessarily. It takes a while for your menstrual cycle to settle down into a regular pattern. *But,* if you've had sex and some ejaculate might have gotten into or even near your vagina, you could be pregnant. Let's go over the possibilities. Suppose you've had sex even once since your last period—then you need to think about these things: Did you or he use an approved contraceptive method *every* time? Which one? If it was a condom, did it slip off or break?

If it was a diaphragm, and you had intercourse twice, did you remember to use an extra application of foam or cream before the second time, *without* removing the diaphragm? Did you leave the diaphragm in for the full eight hours after the last ejaculation? Was it around the fourteenth to the seventeenth day following the first day of your previous period?

If your period still does not start within two weeks after it should have, then you'll feel better—and so will I—if you check with a gynecologist or Planned Parenthood center.

Why do girls have to take it easy when they have a period?

Where did you hear that? It's an old-fashioned idea people used to have that women were weak, fragile creatures. Of course, in those days poor women were working just as hard as men—as they still do. Girls can be as active during a period as at any other time.

What is menopause?

Menopause is the time when a woman stops menstruating. It usually occurs between age forty-five and fifty-five. Menopause may happen almost overnight or it may take several years, during which the woman will have periods at less regular times. After she stops completely, she can no longer become pregnant.

Why do my breasts hurt all the time? How soon will they stop hurting?

They're beginning to grow, so you're getting what we call breast buds. In a couple of months they'll stop hurting but they will keep on growing. Bring me the baby oil and I'll show you how to rub them very gently with your fingers—that should make them feel better.

Are there exercises that will make my breasts bigger?

No, there aren't. The size of your breasts mostly depends on heredity. Think about your mother and your father's sister and mother: Your breasts will probably turn out to be somewhere in that range. They may get a little larger with pregnancy and nursing, or if you gain a lot of weight. Just like the other parts of our bodies, breasts come in all sizes and shapes and no particular one is any better or worse than any other. Certainly women with small breasts can nurse babies as well as large-breasted women. All bodies are beautiful in some way, and we can all learn how to appreciate our best points.

My balls are getting bigger! Am I getting cancer?

No! You're just beginning the changes of puberty. Now you can start watching for pubic hair, then your penis will get longer and thicker and your voice will start to change. About a year and a half to two years from now, you will probably have your first ejaculation.

Why are so many girls my age taller than me?

That may be temporary, because they've already started the spurt of growth that comes at puberty and you haven't begun it yet. Girls tend to start their growth spurt a little sooner than boys do, but don't worry, the boys start to grow before long.

What is a nocturnal emission (wet dream)? Is it okay if I don't have any?

A nocturnal emission is an ejaculation during your sleep that you aren't even aware of until you wake up. It's often called a "wet dream." Having one simply means that your supply of semen has been building up and the wet dream is nature's way of releasing the tension due to that buildup. *Not* having one usually means that you've been releasing the tension by masturbating when you feel sexy. Either way everything's okay.

Can you have a wet dream when you're awake?

No, you can't, because it's a dream. It is possible that some boys can have a sexual daydream and become so involved in their fantasy that they have an ejaculation.

What is a virgin?

Someone who has never had intercourse. For a girl or a woman, that means she has never had a penis inside her vagina. For a boy, it means his penis has never been inside a vagina.

Can a doctor tell if you're a virgin?

In boys, there is probably no way. Young girls have a membrane called the hymen, that covers the vaginal opening. If it is still whole, chances are you are a virgin. However, some girls were born without a hymen, and many girls had their hymens opened during athletics or minor accidents. Many girls have a very elastic hymen, and a penis can enter it without tearing. Of course, using tampons or fingers in the vagina for pleasuring can stretch the hymen. The answer is that nobody could tell for sure if you're a virgin.

Can a virgin use tampons?

Yes. They come in several sizes and anyone can use them.

Are tampons safe?

Many women have used them without difficulty. However, there have been some cases of women using tampons during their periods and then getting an illness called Toxic Shock Syndrome. We don't know enough about the illness or its connection with tampons to be absolutely sure they caused the disease, but, at least for the time being, a lot of women are using sanitary napkins sometimes and tampons other times, instead of relying completely on tampons. Also using smaller size tampons and changing them often is a good idea.

Is "wet dream" another term for masturbation?

No. Masturbation is under conscious control, but a wet dream is involuntary and happens during sleep.

Does a wet dream always come from sex?

Not necessarily. It may happen from an exciting or fearful dream as well as an erotic one.

Can a boy control wet dreams or do they just happen on a regular basis?

No, to both questions. Wet dreams are involuntary, but boys who masturbate frequently seldom or never have them.

Is there any way I can make my penis bigger?

No, none at all. Anyhow, yours is about average size already. Remember, though, penis size doesn't make any difference for the important things like intercourse. A vagina accommodates itself easily to any size penis.

After the testicles mature does sperm come out every time you urinate?

No. Sperm comes out *only* when you have an erection and ejaculate. Just as you cannot urinate while you have an erection, you cannot ejaculate when you urinate.

Why do kids get acne but not grownups?

Acne is a skin eruption that seems to get worse when the hormone balance is disturbed in some way. The balance in your hormones is changing. Because you're becoming an adult very quickly, you have more of some hormones than you did as a child. Most teenagers and some adults have acne. Acne has nothing to do with masturbation or with not being clean, although if you don't wash your face carefully and regularly, it may get worse. Most cases can be treated easily at home; if you like, I'll help you get instructions on how to do this, and if the acne gets too bad we'll be sure to take care of it.

Why don't I ejaculate? John did when he was ten and Billy when he was twelve and I'm almost fourteen and haven't yet. What's wrong with me?

Not a thing. You're just later on the normal time scale than John, who began early, or Billy, who was close to the middle. I know it's hard to wait, but it all evens out, really. When your penis gets longer and thicker, that means you'll probably ejaculate within a few months.

What is a pelvic exam?

That's when a doctor looks into the vagina with a light so that he or she can see the cervix and all parts of the vagina to make sure they are healthy. Then he or she puts a rubber glove on one hand (to avoid bringing any infection into the vagina), inserts the index and middle fingers into the vagina and pushes gently as far as they will go. There they can feel the cervix, which should be firm and smooth. Those two fingers then push upward while the doctor places his or her hand flat on the abdomen below the bellybutton and pushes gently downward toward the fingers inside. That way he or she can feel the uterus and then the ovaries between the fingers of the two hands. If the tissues are healthy they are soft, so he or she can just feel the outlines of the uterus and the ovaries, and judge their size, softness or hardness. This examination should be done regularly throughout a woman's life.

Is it all right for the doctor to touch my genitals?

A doctor who is doing a thorough physical exam should be making sure that every part of your body is healthy, and so he or she *must* use the sense of touch, including touching your genitals. It's a different kind of touching than to give or receive pleasure.

He or she should not be touching your genitals to produce pleasure in you. If you feel he or she is examining you in a non-professional manner, you should ask the doctor to stop. Then you should tell either your parent or some other adult you trust about what happened.

Is it okay to think about sexy things when I masturbate?

Yes, most people do have sexual fantasies then. Fantasies are simply a way of thinking about things that you have done, or expect to do or would like to try, or feel curious about and are trying to imagine even though you might not really want to do them.

Fantasy even makes it possible to imagine doing impossible things. Best of all, fantasies are safe, because they don't have to be made to come true.

Will it hurt if I masturbate four or five times in a row?

No, it can't hurt either boys or girls to masturbate as often as they feel like it. Your body knows when it's time to take a rest and it will tell you so by not feeling good anymore if you go on trying.

Can a boy shoot off (ejaculate) without touching his penis?

Yes. This can happen during intense excitement, like while dancing or sitting close to a girl in a car or while watching something that is sexually arousing. Or it can happen at a moment of great fear, like in a car crash.

For boys: **Does a boy have to shoot his sperm before he can get his penis small again?**

For girls: **Does a girl have to have an orgasm for her clitoris to get soft again?**

No. Usually the erection will go away by itself, unless the penis (clitoris) is rubbed or stimulated. That happens if you stop thinking about sex or become involved in some other activity or are interrupted while you're masturbating or having intercourse.

Do women ever ejaculate?

Yes, a few women do. We know that women's vaginas get wet when they are thinking about sex or when they are excited about it.

That's called lubrication and we used to think that was the only fluid involved in sex for women. Recently, though, we've begun to understand that women may also ejaculate, though it's usually less noticeable than when men do. Women find it very pleasurable when a place in the vagina called the Grafenberg spot (G-spot) is stimulated. Their tissues swell, and when they have an orgasm they may occasionally ejaculate a fluid from the urethra that is very much like semen.

Is an orgasm during intercourse the same as one you get when you are masturbating?

The way that it happens is actually the same for all orgasms, but that doesn't mean they all necessarily *feel* the same. You probably already know how different climax can be from one time to another when you masturbate. It's that way for everybody. You'll discover that there is also the same wide range with intercourse. Some people do feel that masturbation climaxes tend to be very intense because, after lots of experience with self-pleasure, they feel more in control of the process than when another person is involved. But, in general, sexually experienced people don't find the differences great. As your body matures you'll learn more about what gives you pleasure.

For boys: **What are "blue balls"?**

For girls: **Why do I feel so much pressure in my pelvis when I've been making out?**

"Blue balls" is a slang term for pain in the testicles that sometimes happens when a man or boy is stimulated for a long time without having an orgasm. A girl or a woman will feel a kind of heaviness or pressure in her pelvis for the same reason. It's not very important or very serious for either a girl or a boy, and the fact that you may be a little uncomfortable should never be used to put pressure on anybody to have sex if he or she doesn't want to. The discomfort can always be relieved by masturbating.

Does a girl always bleed the first time she makes love?

No. Some girls who have unbroken hymens may bleed a little the first time a penis or fingers are inserted into the vagina. However, if the girl has been using tampons or has been fairly athletic, and if the insertion is gentle, the chances are that she won't bleed.

Can a boy get an erection while he's dancing?

Yes, it happens quite often.

Jimmy is two years younger than me but he says if we "did it" I would have a baby. That isn't true, is it?

Age doesn't have anything to do with it. If the boy has already ejaculated and the girl has already menstruated or is even close to it, then yes, it could be true. Lots of kids have learned this when they tried having intercourse before finding out the facts, and the girl became pregnant. It can happen even to really young girls.

How big does a penis get during intercourse?

On the average a penis swells up to about six inches in length. Some get longer, some shorter, some thicker, some thinner, in all combinations. There is no way to tell by looking at it when it is soft how large a penis will be when it is hard. The differences don't matter anyway, because the vagina is like a long balloon before you blow into it: It can stretch just enough to fit closely around whatever size penis enters it.

Does intercourse hurt the woman?

No, as long as the woman wants it and isn't forced and doesn't tighten up the walls of the vagina against it. That's why it is important for both partners to have loving interaction before intercourse. This way the woman gets aroused gradually, and her vagina becomes well lubricated. Then the penis will enter easily.

How long does intercourse last?

As long or as short a time as the people involved want it to last—often at least until each has had an orgasm. Sometimes some people have intercourse for an hour, or repeatedly over several hours, but something less than thirty minutes is probably more usual.

Is intercourse habit-forming?

Not in the sense that people can become ill if they don't have it regularly. But it is very enjoyable and a very intense way of communicating feelings for a partner, so people like to do it a lot.

What is oral sex?

Oral sex means pleasuring a man by sucking his penis or pleasuring a woman by licking or sucking her clitoris or vulva. The technical term for sucking male genitals is fellatio, for female genitals, cunnilingus. There are a lot of slang words for this kind of pleasuring, and most of them are negative or insulting. You will hear words like "blow job," "going down," or "giving head," but they are not terms that most people want to hear.

Is it okay to go all the way with oral sex or is that just to get ready for intercourse?

Whichever you and your partner prefer.

Can you have intercourse before you have sperm?

Yes, you can.

If two people don't have VD can they get it from having intercourse with each other?

Definitely not. Like any other contagious disease, such as measles or mumps, you can only get a *sexually* transmitted disease from someone who already has it.

Do you get VD from doing it wrong?

No. The only way you can get a sexually transmitted disease is to have sexual contact with someone who is already infected with the disease.

Can you get VD from masturbating or just from intercourse?

You cannot get a sexually transmitted disease from masturbating yourself, but it might be possible for someone else to transfer disease germs from their genitals to yours by first masturbating themselves and then you, especially if you are both female. It is not just intercourse that can transmit a sexual disease; you can also get it from almost any kind of sexual contact with someone who already has it.

How do STDs affect you?

Some involve mostly localized symptoms around the genital area such as sores, itching and abnormal discharge or difficulty in urinating. These are very irritating and may make sex extremely painful. Others may have serious long-term effects on the entire body, causing blindness, mental problems, heart disease, sterility, having an affected baby, or death. It is very important to check with a doctor or a health clinic if you suspect you may have something wrong. And, if there's any question, it's really urgent to let your sexual partner know about it so he or she can also get treatment.

Can sex diseases be cured?

Except for herpes, for which no permanent cure has been found, most sexually transmitted diseases can be cured, but if they are not found and treated early enough, some can leave damage behind that cannot be fixed.

What is a diaphragm?

It is a small, round piece of soft rubber that has to be fitted by a doctor. It is inserted into the vagina and pushed up to block the cervix so that sperm can't get past it. It is *always* used with contraceptive jelly placed inside it and around the edges to make a good seal. It must not be removed from the vagina until eight hours after intercourse in order to prevent the sperm from reaching the egg. It is a very effective way to keep from having a baby, and is also very safe for people's health.

What is a condom (rubber)?

It is a sheath that covers the penis when it is hard and keeps the sperm from getting into the vagina. Most condoms are made of thin rubber. You can buy them easily in the drugstore. If, at the same time, the woman uses a spermicidal (sperm-killing) jelly, cream or foam, this makes the method much more effective than the condom alone. A condom can also be used for extra protection when a woman is ovulating, even though she is using a diaphragm.

What is the Pill?

It is a hormone the woman takes every day to keep her ovaries from producing any eggs. Of course, if there are no eggs, she can't have a baby. It is a very effective method, but doctors don't feel it's at all safe for young girls to use. Some older women also feel that taking the Pill every day isn't very healthy for their bodies. Some people like it because it is so effective, but there are a lot of questions about being "on the Pill," which is the way people usually describe this method. People who use the Pill should be examined regularly by a doctor who is watching for side-effects.

What is the IUD?

It is a small bit of plastic, often "S" shaped, with a little string tied to the end. The doctor puts it into the uterus through the cervix. It keeps a fertilized egg from attaching itself to the wall of the uterus so that it can't develop into a baby. The little string hangs out through the cervix into the vagina, where the woman can regularly feel it to make certain the IUD is still there. Some people have used an IUD for a long time, others have had trouble with it. Young women should never use the IUD because it has caused a lot of health problems in this age group.

What is a cervical cap?

It is a small cap-shaped piece of solid rubber, plastic or gold that is custom-fitted by a doctor to fit over a woman's cervix—the bottom part of the uterus that sticks down into the vagina. The cervix is the entrance through which the sperm get up into the uterus and eventually to the egg; the cap blocks the opening of the cervix. Correctly used, it is as effective as the diaphragm, and can be left in place for several days. Unfortunately, not all physicians know how to fit it properly.

What does "abortion" mean?

Abortion means that a fetus that was formed when a sperm and an egg got together does not develop into a baby who can live outside the mother's uterus. Sometimes—usually because there's something wrong with the pregnancy—the fetus comes out through the vagina by itself. This is called a spontaneous abortion or a miscarriage.

Sometimes, if she finds herself pregnant and she has a serious illness, or she feels she cannot be a good mother at this time of her life, a woman decides to have an abortion—to have the fetus removed from her uterus by a doctor. Almost everybody feels sad when a pregnancy has to be stopped, but most people feel a woman should have the right to decide about that since she can best judge what would be best for her and the baby. Other people, though, are very much against abortion and are trying to have the law changed to prevent it. Several religious groups feel that way, too. It's a hard and complicated question for everyone, and it would be good for people always to use the most effective birth-control methods when they have intercourse, to avoid an unwanted pregnancy.

What's a queer?

"Queer" is an insulting word that some people use for a homosexual. It's just as bad as calling a black person a nigger, or a Jewish person a kike or an Italian person a wop. They are all insults, and when someone talks that way we call it bigotry, which is being intolerant of people who are different from you. Bigots are often cruel to homosexuals, and can make their lives unnecessarily unhappy.

What is a transsexual?

A man (or less often a woman) may decide to have a series of operations to change from one sex to the other, including changing the genitals. The man would then say he *is* a woman, and wants to be treated like a woman. This is called a transsexual operation, and the person who has it done is called a transsexual. You sometimes read in the paper about people who have had this operation; usually they feel very strongly that they really are a member of the other sex, born into the wrong body. That's why they want to make the change.

If I get a hard-on when I'm around a certain boy, does that mean I'm gay?

Perhaps, but not necessarily. Boys get crushes on other boys sometimes, as well as on girls. Girls also can admire, love and be turned on by boys and also by girls. People who consider themselves gay usually have a clear preference for other persons of the same sex.

What is sodomy?

Sodomy is the legal term for having anal intercourse. Many people, heterosexual as well as homosexual, have this kind of intercourse, which involves placing the penis in the anus.

Are gay men always effeminate?

Not at all. They include the same range of types as heterosexuals, including professional football players, artists, truck drivers, musicians and policemen. By the same token, gay women, or lesbians, are no different from other women and may prefer to dress and act in traditional "feminine" ways or to dress and act with fewer frills.

How come some homosexuals are married?

Probably very few people who are exclusively homosexual get married. More likely they are bisexual—that is, interested in both sexes. People like this often marry in order to have children. Because our society makes it pretty rough for bisexuals or declared homosexuals, most people want to live what looks like a "normal" life. But of course it's very hard to keep such an important part of your life a secret.

If gay people raise a child, will the child be gay too?

Usually not. There's about the same likelihood for the child of a gay parent to be gay as for the child of a straight parent.

What does it mean to "come out of the closet"?

Many homosexuals feel that they have to hide the way they live, and the persons they love, because so many people in our society are cruel to them. But that makes them feel that they are concealing an important part of themselves—because loving someone is one of the biggest parts of our lives. So they may decide that, whatever the bigots might do, they want to be honest in the world, and they start saying, "I'm a homosexual," or "I'm gay," or "I'm a lesbian." This is called "coming out of the closet."

What is a vasectomy?

That is male sterilization, the man's version of a woman's having her tubes tied. The doctor cuts a short piece out of the vas on both sides. These are the two tubes that carry sperm from the testicles, where they are manufactured. The four cut ends of the tubes are either burned with a small electric current or closed by one of several other methods. The result permanently prevents sperm from getting into the seminal fluid, so the man can no longer make a woman pregnant. The operation is simple and doesn't hurt. The testicles still produce sperm, but they just get absorbed into the man's body fluids and disappear.

Male sterilization has no effect on sexual pleasure. The semen looks the same to the naked eye, and both sex drive and ejaculation remain the same.

What does "having your tubes tied" mean?

That is female sterilization, and does the same thing as a vasectomy for men. The Fallopian tube is cut or blocked surgically so no ovum (egg) can go down it into the uterus or get fertilized by a sperm. Usually the operation can't be reversed, so before she has the procedure done a woman needs to be certain that she doesn't want any more children for the rest of her life. Female sterilization has no effect on sexual pleasure or sex drive.

OTHER BOOKS FOR
YOUR FAMILY TO SHARE

One of the best ways to encourage open conversation about sex with your family is to have books on the subject around the house, easily accessible to everyone, regardless of age. Remember that children are not hurt by exposure to what may seem to you like information too advanced for their age: If they don't need it at the moment, they simply pass it by. Later, when they do need that information, they'll know where to find it.

The books on the following list have been carefully selected for different ages and different special needs.

READING LIST

For Children—Arranged from Youngest to Oldest

How Babies Are Made, by Andrew C. Andry and Steven Schepp. The story of reproduction in plants, animals and humans, told through color photographs of paper sculptures. Factually accurate and easily understood. (New York: Time-Life, Inc., 1968.)

Did the Sun Shine before You Were Born: A Sex Education Primer, by Sol Gordon and Judith Cohen. A book parents can read with their children, describing how different kinds of families live and grow. (New York: Okpaku Communications, 1977.)

How Was I Born? A Photographic Story of Reproduction and Birth for Children, by Lennart Nilsson. To read aloud. Tells the story of reproduction and birth, using the famous Nilsson photographs of fetal development in combination with warm family scenes and other illustrations. (New York: Delacorte Press, 1975.)

Love and Sex and Growing Up, by Corinne Benson Johnson and Eric W. Johnson. Deals with many topics to help elementary-age children think about being a man or a woman, and what this means. (Paper: New York: Bantam Books, Inc., 1979.)

Period, by JoAnn Gardner-Loulan, Bonnie Lopez and Marcia Quackenbush. Reassuring, cleverly illustrated book about menstruation. Explains why all girls are normal, yet each one is special. (Rev. ed.; San Francisco: New Glide Publications, 1981.)

Love and Sex in Plain Language, by Eric W. Johnson. Basic information on sexuality, emphasizing that it should always be seen in the context of one's total personality and expressed in responsible, respectful, caring relationships. (3rd rev. ed.; New York: Harper & Row, Inc., 1979. Paper: New York: Bantam Books, Inc., 1974.)

Facts about Sex for Today's Youth, by Sol Gordon. A short, direct approach covers anatomy, reproduction, love and sex questions. Gives definitions, including slang terms. Well illustrated. (Paper: rev. ed., Fayetville: Ed-U Press, 1979.)

Learning about Sex: The Contemporary Guide for Young Adults, by Gary F. Kelly. This book, while giving basic factual information, focuses on attitudes and the process of making sexual decisions responsibly. (Woodbury: Barron's Educational Series, Inc., 1977.)

For Families

The Family Book about Sexuality, by Mary S. Calderone and Eric W. Johnson. Illustrated by Vivien Cohen. A comprehensive approach to the family's understanding of the sexuality and sexual concerns of all of its members. (New York: Harper & Row, Inc., 1981. Paper: New York: Bantam Books, Inc., 1983.)

Sex: The Facts, The Acts, and Your Feelings, by Michael Carrera. Comprehensive, in-depth, easy-to-understand information about sexuality presented in a nonjudgmental tone, but imparting values concerning people and relationships. (New York: Crown Publishers, 1981.)

On Becoming a Family: The Growth of Attachment, by T. Berry Brazelton. In this wonderful book for all parents and especially for the parent-to-be, a well-known pediatrician reveals how the bonds between parents and baby are developed and deepened. (New York: Delacorte, 1981. Paper: New York: Dell Publishing Co., Inc., 1981.)

Special Subjects

Growing Up Free: Raising Your Kids in the 80's, by Letty Cottin Pogrebin. Child-rearing from conception to puberty, emphasizing nonsexist sex education, parity parenting and gender-neutral attitudes. (New York: McGraw-Hill, Inc., 1980. Paper: New York: Bantam Books, Inc., 1981.)

Now That You Know: What Every Parent Should Know about Homosexuality, by Betty Fairchild and Betty Hayward. Informative, sensitively written guide for parents of homosexual children, but equally helpful for all parents, whose children will eventually want to understand their homosexual friends. (Paper: Harcourt Brace Jovanovich, 1981.)

VD—And What You Should Do about It, by Eric W. Johnson. For any age; facts simply given, but no "horror" pictures. (New, revised edition. Harper & Row, Inc., 1978.)

Sex without Shame: Encouraging the Child's Healthy Sexual Development, by Alayne Yates. Explains primary facts about how children's sexuality develops and what parents can do to help. (New York: William Morrow and Co., Inc., 1978.)

BIBLIOGRAPHY

The confidence and competence with which a book on sex for parents and children can be written must rest on the research findings of many scientists. The following are among those to whom we are indebted for the light their work has shed on the sexual lives of children.

Aries, P. *Centuries of Childhood: A Social History of Family Life* (New York: Vintage Books, 1962).

Ash, M. "The Misnamed Female Sex Organ," in *Childhood and Sexuality*. Proceedings of the International Symposium, Montreal, Quebec, September 7–9, 1979 (Montreal: Editions Etudes Vivantes, 1980).

Bandura, A. and R. H. Walters. *Social Learning and Personality Development* (New York: Holt, Rinehart and Winston, 1963).

Bernstein, A. C. and P. A. Cowan. "Children's Concepts of How People Get Babies," in *Childhood and Sexuality*. Proceedings of the International Symposium, Montreal, Quebec, September 7–9, 1979 (Montreal: Editions Etudes Vivantes, 1980).

Blackman, N. "Pleasure and Touching," in *Childhood and Sexuality*. Proceedings of the International Symposium, Montreal, Quebec, September 7–9, 1979 (Montreal: Editions Etudes Vivantes, 1980).

Broderick, C. B. and S. E. Fowler. "New Patterns of Relationships between the Sexes among Preadolescents." *Marriage and Family Living*, 23:1 (February 1961).

Broderick, C. and G. P. Rowe. "A Scale of Preadolescent Heterosexual Development." *Journal of Marriage and the Family* 30 (February 1968).

Cohen, B. and S. Parker. "Sex Information among Nursery School Children," in Oremland, E. K., and J. Oremland (eds.), *The Sexual and Gender Development of Young Children: The Role of the Educator* (Cambridge, Mass.: Ballinger, 1977).

Conn, J. H. "Children's Reactions to the Discovery of Genital Differences." *The American Journal of Orthopsychiatry* 10 (1940).

Drake, L. W., C. Nederlander and R. G. Mercier. "Teaching Sexual Assertiveness Training: Sex Education between Parent and Child," in *Childhood and Sexuality*. Proceedings of the International Symposium, Montreal, Quebec, September 7–9, 1979 (Montreal: Editions Etudes Vivantes, 1980).

Elias, J. and P. Gebhard. "Sexuality and Sexual Learning in Children." *Phi Delta Kappen* 50 (March 1969).

Erikson, E. "The Problem of Ego Identity," in Stein, M., et al., *Identity and Anxiety* (Glencoe, Ill.: Free Press, 1960).

Finch, S. M. "Sex Play among Boys and Girls." *Medical Aspects of Human Sexuality* (September 1969).

Finkelhor, D. "The Sexual Climate in Families." Paper presented at Family Sexuality Conference, University of Minnesota Medical School, Minneapolis, Minn., June 3, 1980.

Gadpaille, W. J. "A Consideration of Two Concepts of Normality as It Applies to Adolescent Sexuality." *Journal of the American Academy of Child Psychiatry* 15 (Autumn 1976).

————. "Critical Sexual Needs in the School Years: What Can Children Not Do Without?" Paper presented at 16th National Conference on Physicians and Schools, sponsored by the American Medical Association, Chicago, Ill., November 9, 1978.

Gagnon, J. H. "Sexuality and Sexual Learning in the Child." *Psychiatry* 28 (August 1965).

————, and C. S. Greenblat. *Life Designs: Individuals, Marriages, and Families* (Glenview, Ill.: Scott, Foresman, & Company, 1978).

————, and W. Simon. *Sexual Conduct: The Social Sources of Human Sexuality* (Chicago: Aldine Press, 1973).

Gesell, A. and F. L. Ilg. *The Child from Five to Ten*. Rev. ed. (New York: Harper and Row, Inc., 1977).

Goldman, R. and J. Goldman. *Children's Sexual Thinking* (Boston, Mass.: Routledge and Keegan Paul, 1982).

Gordon, S., P. Scales and K. Everly. *The Sexual Adolescent* (North Scituate, Mass.: Duxbury, 1979).

Gripton, J. "Preparing Parents for Participating in the Sexual Development of Their Children: An Innovative Program and a Research Design." *Childhood and Sexuality.* Proceedings of the International Symposium, Montreal, Quebec, September 7–9, 1979 (Montreal: Editions Etudes Vivantes, 1980).

Guttmacher Institute. *11 Million Teenagers: What Can Be Done about the Epidemic of Adolescent Pregnancies in the United States* (New York: Planned Parenthood Federation of America, 1976).

Halverson, H. M. "Genital and Sphincter Behavior of the Male Infant." *Journal of Genetic Psychology* 56 (1940).

Ilg, F. L. et al. *Child Behavior.* Rev. ed. (New York: Harper and Row, 1981).

Ketcher, A. "The Discrimination of Sex Differences by Young Children." *Journal of Genetic Psychology* 87 (1955).

Kinsey, A. C., W. B. Pomeroy and C. E. Martin. *Sexual Behavior in the Human Male* (Philadelphia: Saunders, 1948).

———— et al. *Sexual Behavior in the Human Female* (Philadelphia: Saunders, 1953).

Klaus, M. and J. Kennell. *Maternal-Infant Bonding: The Impact of Early Separation or Loss on Family Development* (St. Louis: C. V. Mosby Company, 1976).

Kreitler, H. S. "Children's Concepts of Sexuality and Birth." *Child Development* 37 (1966).

Laing, R. D. *Knots* (New York: Pantheon Books, 1970).

Langfeldt, T. "Sexual Development in Children," in M. Cook and K. Howells (eds.), *Adult Sexual Interest in Children* (London: Academic Press, 1980).

Lewis, M. and J. Kagan. "Studies in Attention." *Merrill-Palmer Quarterly* II (1965).

Maddock, J. W. "Sex in Adolescence: Its Meaning and Future." *Adolescence* 8 (1973).

Martinson, F. M. *Infant and Child Sexuality* (St. Peter, Minn.: Gustafus Aldolpus College, 1973).

Masters, W. H. and V. E. Johnson. "The Role of Religion in Sexual Dysfunction," in M. S. Calderone (ed.), *Sexuality and Human Values* (New York: Association Press, 1974).

Mead, M. and M. Wolfenstein (eds.). *Childhood in Contemporary Cultures* (Chicago: University of Chicago Press, 1963).

Mohr, J. W., R. E. Turner and M. B. Jerry. *Pedophilia and Exhibitionism* (Toronto: University of Toronto Press, 1964).

Money, J. and H. Musaph (eds.). *Handbook of Sexology*, Vols. I, II, III and IV (North Holland: Elsevier, 1977).

Morrison, E. S. et al. *Growing Up Sexual* (New York: Van Nostrand Company, 1980).

Newson, J. and E. Newson. *Four Years Old in an Urban Community* (Chicago: Aldine, 1968).

Peller, L. "Sex Education of the Young Child." *Journal of Sex Research* I (March 1965).

Rainwater, L. *Behind Ghetto Walls: Black Families in a Federal Slum* (Chicago: Aldine, 1970).

Ramey, J. W. "Preadolescent Sexuality." Keynote Address, Department of Health, Education and Welfare Conference on Preadolescent Sexuality, Mt. Washington, N.H., October, 1977.

————. "Positive Socialization of Incestuous Desires." Plenary Address: Family Sexuality Conference, University of Minnesota Medical School, Minneapolis, Minn., June 2, 1980.

Ramsey, G. V. "The Sexual Development of Boys." *American Journal of Psychology* 56 (1943).

————. "The Sex Information of Younger Boys." *The American Journal of Orthopsychiatry*, 13 (April 1943).

Reevy, W. R. "Child Sexuality," in Ellis, A. and Abarbanel (eds.), *The Encyclopedia of Sexual Behavior* (New York: Hawthorn Books, Inc., 1967).

Roberts, E. J. and S. A. Holt. "Parent-Child Communication about Sexuality." *SIECUS Report* VIII, #4 (March 1980).

Rutter, M. "Normal Psychosexual Development." *Journal of Child Psychiatry* 11 (1971).

Sears, R., E. Macoby and A. Levin. *Patterns of Child Rearing* (New York: Harper and Row, 1957).

Segel, J. (ed.). *The Mental Health of the Child* (Washington, D.C.: Public Health Service Publication #2168, 1971).

Secondi, J. J. *For People Who Make Love: A Doctor's Guide to Sexual Health* (New York: Taplinger Publishing Company, 1975).

Siegel, A. "Long-term Outcomes of Early Childhood Experiences." (Paper prepared for the Project on Human Sexual Development, 1975.)

Solnit, A. J. "Sexual and Gender Development in the Context of the Family, School and Society," in E. K. Oremland and J. Oremland (eds.), *The Sexual and Gender Development of Young Children: The Role of the Educator* (Cambridge, Mass.: Ballinger, 1977).

Sorensen, R. C. *Adolescent Sexuality in Contemporary America* (New York: World Publishing, 1973).

Spitz, R. A. "Autoeroticism Re-examined: The Role of Early Sexual Behavior Patterns in Personality Formation." *The Psychoanalytic Study of the Child* 17:183–315 (New York: International University Press, 1962).

Tiefer, L. *Human Sexuality, Feelings and Functions* (New York: Harper and Row, 1979).

Vanggaard, T. *Phallos* (London: Johathan Cape, 1972), in T. Langfeldt, "Sexual Development in Children," in M. Cook and K. Howells (eds.), *Adult Sexual Interest in Children* (London: Academic Press, 1980).

Yates, A. *Sex without Shame: Encouraging the Child's Healthy Sexual Development* (New York: Morrow, 1978).

————. "The Effect of Commonly Accepted Parenting Practices on Erotic Development," in *Childhood and Sexuality*. Proceedings of the International Symposium, Montreal, Quebec, September 7–9, 1979 (Montreal: Editions Etudes Vivantes, 1980).

INDEX

ABOUT THE AUTHORS

One of the world's leading experts in sex education, MARY STEICHEN CALDERONE, M.D., is a former medical director of the Planned Parenthood Federation of America. She was co-founder and president of SIECUS (Sex Information and Education Council of the U.S.) from 1964 to 1982, and is now adjunct professor at New York University, in the Human Sexuality Program of its Department of Health Education. She is a charter member of the American College of Sexologists.

JAMES W. RAMEY, ED. D., is a behavioral scientist specializing in biomedical research and is a member of the American College of Sexologists. He is the author of many articles and several books, including *Intimate Friendships* and *Television in Medical Education and Research*. He was executive director of the Institute for Advancement of Medical Communication, Senior Research Associate, Center for Policy Research, and visiting professor, Bowman Gray School of Medicine. Dr. Ramey now devotes his time to writing.